T0205908

SpringerBriefs in Statistics

More information about this series at http://www.springer.com/series/8921

Jamalludin Ab Rahman

Brief Guidelines for Methods and Statistics in Medical Research

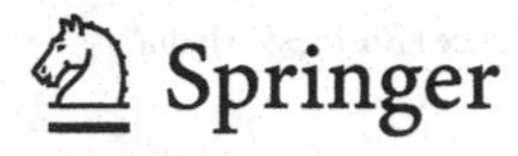

Jamalludin Ab Rahman
Department of Community Medicine,
Kulliyyah of Medicine
International Islamic University Malaysia
Kuantan, Pahang
Malaysia

ISSN 2191-544X ISSN 2191-5458 (electronic)
SpringerBriefs in Statistics
ISBN 978-981-287-923-3 ISBN 978-981-287-925-7 (eBook)
DOI 10.1007/978-981-287-925-7

Library of Congress Control Number: 2015951348

Springer Singapore Heidelberg New York Dordrecht London

Printed on acid-free paper

Springer Science+Business Media Singapore Pte Ltd. is part of Springer Science+Business Media (www.springer.com)

Preface

Those doing research should agree that both knowledge and understanding on research methodology and statistical analysis are essential and critical. So this book combines both disciplines at one place. The aim is to provide guidelines on how to plan and conduct research in medicine and health care. It is suitable for students and medical or healthcare practitioners with relevant examples and data used. There are already many books on research methodology available in the circulation. There are also many biostatistics books with step-by-step instruction using SPSS. This book is not meant to repeat all information from those books but rather to complement them. Only critical points are mentioned in the book making it a good option for a quick reference on research methodology. Important and critical points are gathered from various sources and from my own experience.

This book is divided into two main parts. Chapter 1 is about research methodology and Chap. 2 is on how to analyse the data. Chapter 1 begins with an overview of how to conduct a research. Emphasis is made for a good understanding of the problem being investigated and how to visualise them graphically. Then the book covers important information about study designs, sampling strategies and sample size calculation. Good data collection starts with a good planning and this is elaborated before the chapter ends with the summary of critical points in research methodology.

Those coming from non-mathematical side often find difficult when it comes to data analysis. So the statistical analysis chapter is written by showing step-by-step format using IBM SPSS Statistics for Windows with some important notes provided when required. Relevant explanation on the results is given with some examples of how to present them for some analyses. Data for the exercise are available at www.jamalrahman.net/book/dataset.

I hope this book will be useful for undergraduates, postgraduates or even professionals in medical research.

June 2015 Jamalludin Ab Rahman

Contents

Chapter 1
Planning a Research

Abstract Research requires sound methodology. It begins by properly identify good research topic, intensive background literatures and clear concept. Objectives are written with SMART criteria. Relevant variables are identified, defined and planned on how they are to be collected in standard manner. Statistical analyses should then be planned in great detail.

Keywords Research methodology · Research design · Sampling · Sample size · Data collection · Validity and reliability · Quality of data

What is research? Literally research means a careful or diligent search; systematic inquiries, investigations or experimentations to discover or to prove theories. In medicine, research is initiated to measure magnitude of diseases, maybe in population or institution; or even among a specific group of people. Research is also conducted to prove how good the new drugs, methods or any invention when compared to the existing ones. Research helps policy makers to design and plan strategies based on best available evidence.

The most important requirement to start a research is to know **why** we would like to conduct one. We may do research to:

- decide the best treatment for patient,
- measure prevalence of a disease in the community,
- determine risk factors for common health problem,
- describe health seeking behaviour in a population,
- prove that the new drug is better than the old one; or for many other reasons.

For every reason above, we need to determine the relevant **variables** involved. Let us assume that we would like to study the prevalence of obesity in our area and its distribution by age, gender, and race. Obesity is the main variable, and we can call it **outcome** variable. Age, gender, and race are the explanatory variables or can be called as **factors**. These variables need to be identified through thorough literature review. They should not be chosen conveniently or haphazardly. Once variables for the research are identified and justified, study design has to be decided and this is based on what one like to achieve. Study to describe the current load of illness is not

J. Ab Rahman, *Brief Guidelines for Methods and Statistics in Medical Research*, SpringerBriefs in Statistics,
DOI 10.1007/978-981-287-925-7_1

the same as to test hypotheses or to determine causality. Different study designs have different strengths and weaknesses. This shall be discussed further in Sect. 1.3.

Next thing to consider is the sampling plan. Technique of sampling and sample size depends on your objective again and on how many sample you could afford in term of time, man power and money. A very important note about sample size is that it is an **estimation** from previous studies and from one own expectation for the final results. Then, researchers need to describe data collection process in detail, starting by selecting and defining all relevant variables. Using the same objective mentioned above, obesity is one of the variable but its definition can be derived from body mass index (BMI), waist circumference (where abdominal obesity is more appropriate), fat percentage of the body or even skin fold thickness. If obesity is defined using BMI, the actual data to be collected are body weight and height. Description of obesity should include information about instruments used to measure weight and height. All data need to be captured either using paper-based forms or electronic devices.

Quality of data collection has to be ensured and supervised. Standard data management and detail plan for data analysis have to be prepared before the actual data collection. The summary of these basic steps in research is described in Fig. 1.1.

1.1 Building Problem Statement

Problem statement summarises the whole study. It sits between what had been done previously and what is expected at the end. Problem statement should be completed after good literature review had been done. But before one could even start searching for information, he must know where to start and what to look for. He must somehow have some idea about the problem. So start with some basic problem statement, search for references and information, then improve the problem statement with the new understanding.

Problem statements should consist *what* is actually the main issue (the problem) that triggers the study, including the reasons (*why*) to conduct the study; and *how* the relationship between variables related to the problem. It should end with a description of the expected outcomes.

How to describe the problem? It is easier to construct a problem statement when we could visualise the relationships between variables. The relationship between an **outcome** and a **factor** (or also called explanatory variable or exposure in many other references) can be simplified as in Fig. 1.2. The use of bubble chart or flow chart is also known as **conceptual framework**.[1]

To illustrate this, we use a simple example, the association between obesity (as outcome) and diet (factor). Obesity should be defined clearly. Obesity can be measured as a dichotomous variable i.e. Yes and No. Yes in this case can be defined

---

[1]Conceptual framework is not a causal diagram but it is useful if causality is integrated in the construction of the diagram especially in quantitative studies.

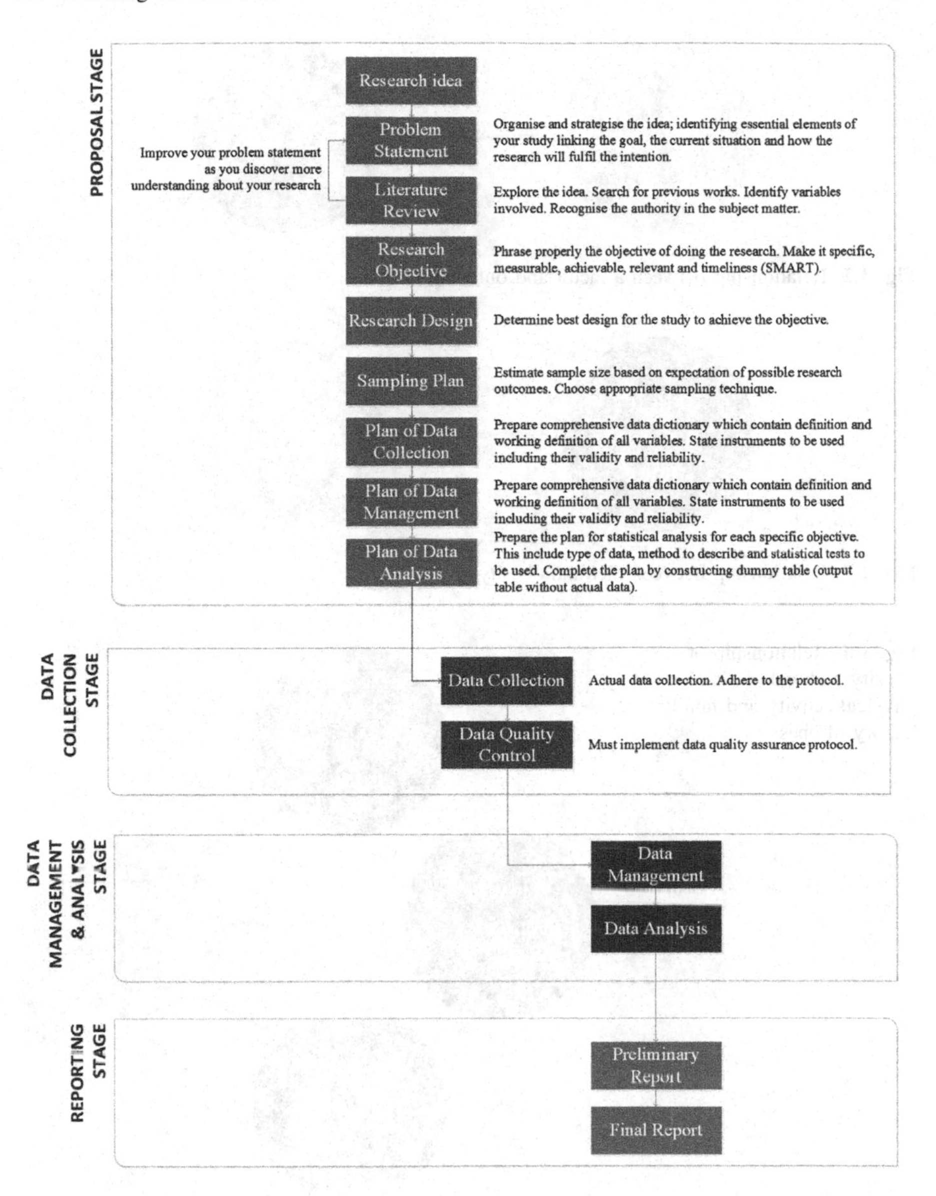

Fig. 1.1 The research plan

when BMI is 30 kg/m^2 or more. Diet can be measured as numerical variables in kCal using 24-h diet recall. The simple logic would be, the higher the kCal intake, the higher the probability of being obese (Fig. 1.3).

However, life is not that simple. There are many factors related to obesity including physical activity, calorie intake, and genetic. Some we can measure directly, some we cannot. Genetic for instance, it is not easy to determine but the presence of obesity in first degree relative would be the easiest proxy albeit not accurate. We may simplify this relationship as in Fig. 1.4.

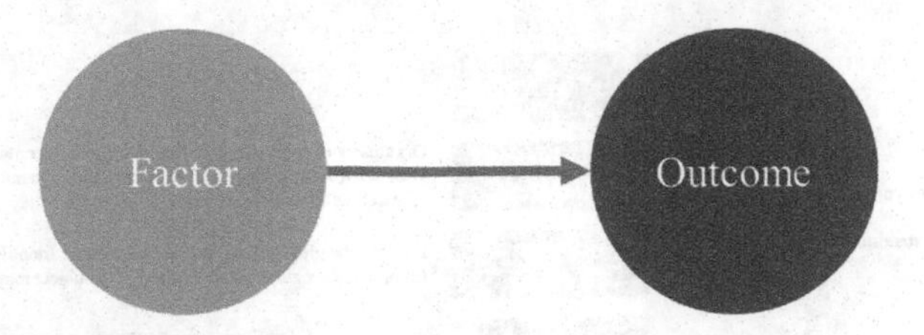

Fig. 1.2 Relationship between a factor and outcome

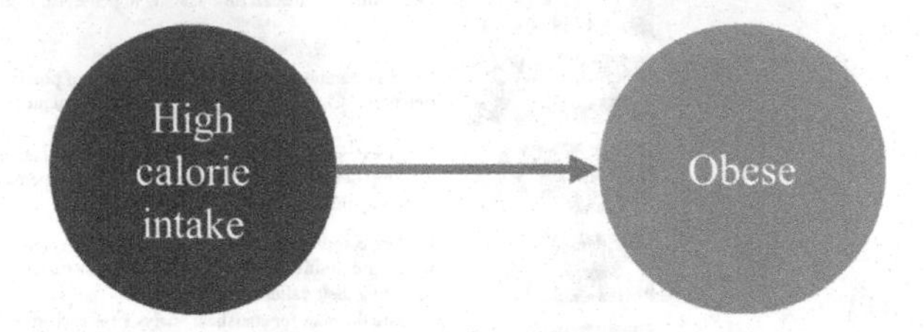

Fig. 1.3 Relationship between diet and obesity

Fig. 1.4 Relationship of obesity with calorie intake, physical activity and family history of obese

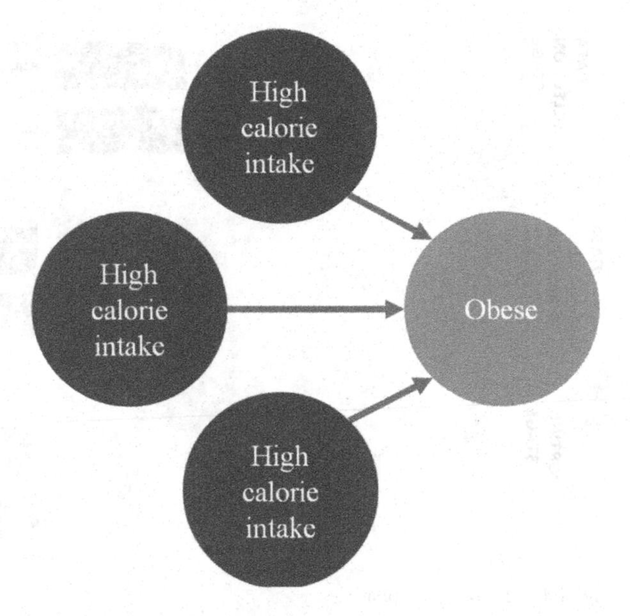

In research even a simple multifactorial relationship like this has to be further defined. Are we trying to ***discover significant factors related to obesity***, or are we trying to ***prove that high calorie intake is independently***[2] ***associated with obesity***

[2]Independent here means, calorie intake is a significant factor related to obesity even after we take into account the influence of other factors such as physical activity and family history. Whether those factors significantly related to obesity or not is not important.

(after we controlled for physical activity and family history). Pause for a while, and read the sentence again. The statistical analysis could be similar but the interpretation is different. In the first statement, we wish to identify factors associated with obesity. The factors can be many. But in the later objective, our interest is on calorie intake and obesity. Physical activity and family history can be identified as confounders. Therefore, it is important to decide which is going to be our objective in order for us to describe the conceptual framework very well.

If the important variables had been identified and their relationship is understood, the construction of problem statement would be easy. However, please be informed that not every research requires complicated statement. More often than not, especially in clinical experiments, we may simply want to prove than the new intervention is better.

1.2 Effective Literature Search

Students often struggle when it comes to doing literature review. This is very common because they are not yet the expert in the field. Therefore, they might not know where to start searching for information and what to look for.

I would like to propose a 5S step in doing *literature* review; *Strategies, Search, Screen, Sort and Summarise* (Fig. 1.5).

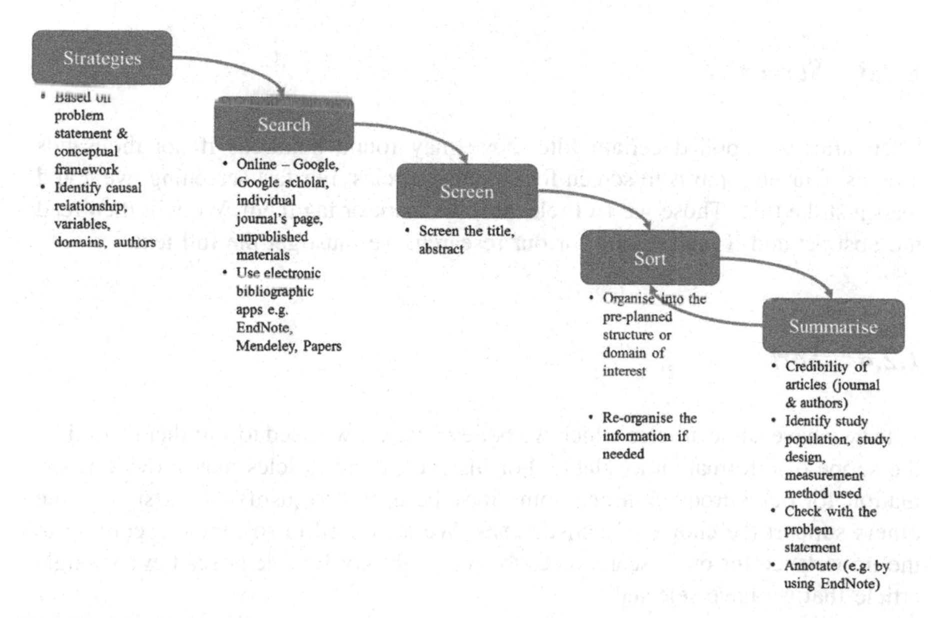

Fig. 1.5 The 5S literature review strategy

1.2.1 Strategies (Planning)

This is the most important step. Literature review would be ***easier if we know what we want from the research***. This is when the conceptual framework or problem statement mentioned above is going to help us. We should identify which are dependent variables, and which are the independent variables. Noting down the authors name and the domain of interest (e.g. epidemiology, therapeutics, diagnostics or prognostics) might further help us to get relevant references. The authority of the subject should be appeared and cited many times.

1.2.2 Search

This is the step where we will do the actual search. These days we usually use online sources such as PubMed Central, Google Scholar or the individual journals' websites e.g. BMJ, Lancet, JAMA etc. We should search using the specific keywords we already discovered in the previous step. We could also search for references using bibliographic manager such as EndNote or Mekentosj Paper. When we search, whether using search engine or application, we should be more specific by applying certain filters. We may limit to recent articles, maybe within the last 5 years only, or limit based on certain study design or even language.

1.2.3 Screen

Even after we applied certain filters, we may found hundreds if not thousands articles. Our next job is to screen for suitable articles. For fast screening, we could read just the title. Those we feel relevant, we mark or tag them. We will then read the abstract and if really good for our research, we must get the full text.

1.2.4 Sort

After we have some articles which we believe useful, we need to sort them based on the scope of information available. For instance, some articles may provide information for our introduction and some may be useful to justify our design, while others support the choice of statistic tests. We also need to sort them according to the importance for our research because we might not be able to read every single article that we have selected.

1.2.5 Summarise

Now it is the time to start reading each of the articles according to the importance. It will become very helpful later if we summarise the article while we are reading them. We may create a table to summarise all these. Jot down the first author's name, year of publication, the design, sample size, instruments, maybe statistical analyses used, and of course the results of the study. After we did the summary, we may need to reorganise the articles again based on the new information acquired.

Good literature search will help us to understand what we really want and what would be our expectation.

1.3 Choosing Best Study Design

Study design can be divided into observational and experimental. Observational means, we only observe the changes. No intervention applied to the samples. Experimental study design means that there will be comparison of effect for different intervention or treatment (Fig. 1.6).

Each design has its strength and weakness and it is important to use best design that suits our research objective (Table 1.1). The most common mistake is using a cross-sectional design to prove causality.

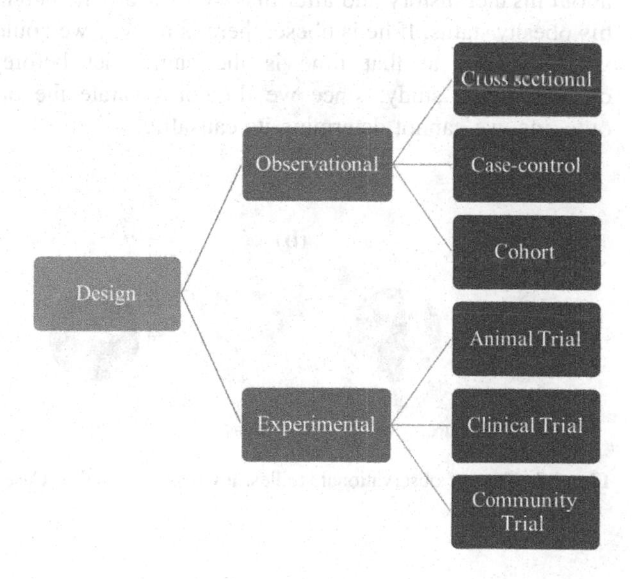

Fig. 1.6 Study design

Table 1.1 Guide in choosing best design

Objective	Cross-sectional	Case-control	Cohort	Experimental
Measure prevalence of disease	++++	−	+	−
Measure incidence of disease	+	−	++++	−
Identify multiple exposures	+	++++	++	+
Identify multiple outcomes	+	−	++++	+
Describe association	+	++	+++	++++
Determine causality	−	+	+++	++++

+ = Recommended, − = Not suitable

1.3.1 Observational Study

Observational study design can be further divided into cross-sectional, case-control and cohort study. Figure 1.7 illustrates the difference concept between the three designs. Most important is to determine what are we measuring (or observing).

1.3.2 Cross-Sectional Study

In cross-sectional study (Fig. 1.7a), we will observe **outcome and factor** at the same time. For example, if we study obesity and diet, we interview a respondent about his diet history and after that we measure the height and weight to determine his obesity status. If he is obese, there is no way we could tell whether the diet that we calculated at that time is the same diet before he becomes obese. In cross-sectional study, since we do not separate the observation of factor from outcome, we cannot determine its causality.

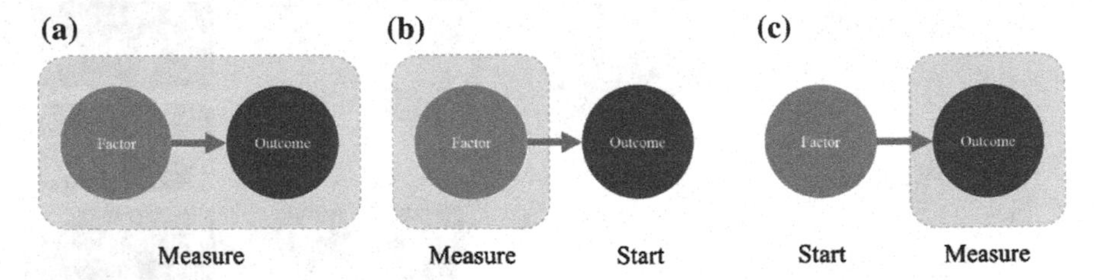

Fig. 1.7 Type of observational studies. **a** Cross-sectional. **b** Case-control. **c** Cohort

1.3.3 Case-Control Study

In case-control study, we will start by having two groups of samples; the case and control. Case is a group with the **outcome** of interest, while control is a group without that characteristic. This means, when the study is initiated the outcomes are already established. If we wish to study factors associated with obesity, case is the group of obese samples and control is the group with normal weight samples. In case-control study, we do not measure or observe the outcomes, but we **measure the factors** (or exposures) associated with it (Fig. 1.7b). This means, the direction of observation is backward. That is why case-control study is a **retrospective** study.[3] In this design, since what we measure is the factor that had occurred previously, we will rely on the **recall** capability of the respondents. We could not analyse the blood or any specimen now to detect historical values. Therefore, case-control study is exposed to some degrees of measurement bias, i.e. recall bias. In case-control study, we already know how many with or without the outcome. Therefore, it is ridiculous to measure the prevalence when we were the one who decide how many samples with and without the outcome of interest.

1.3.4 Cohort Study

Cohort is a prospective study design. The direction of observation is always forward. That means we **measure the outcomes** (Fig. 1.7c). We will start from one time and follow up the respondent (or usually called participants) into the future, observing for any outcome of interest. We can either start from the present time or we can start historically. The latter is known as retrospective cohort study. The most important requirement for a cohort study is that the participants should be free from the outcome at the beginning (inception) of the study. Using the same hypothetical example, if the aim is to determine causes for obesity, we should start the study among non-obese participants. We follow them up over some reasonable times. If we have specific exposures we like to relate to obesity, we can even split the participants into group with exposure of interest, and those without it.

As an example, we may want to study the effect of sedentary lifestyle and its effect to body weight. So we could purposely recruit non-obese participants with sedentary lifestyle, and other non-obese participants who have active lifestyle. We can compare those working in office versus those working at construction sites. At the end of certain period, for example after 10 years, we may compare the weight. We than compare how many from those office workers become obese, and how many those working in construction become obese. However, in that 10 years' time, some of the participants might move out from town and maybe some refuse to be

[3]Do not confuse retrospective study with study that is using old record. Retrospective means the observation is backward, not because the source of data is historical. Source of data has nothing to do with study design. One can still do cross-sectional study using hospital records.

followed up. This is the common disadvantage of a cohort study; loss to follow up (attrition). There is also a possibility that some office workers change their occupation. Same goes to those labours. If the problem is not serious and not many, we can drop the participants from the group and compare only those remaining.

Cohort study is able to show causal relationship because it has temporal association. We start with a group of people without the outcome; we follow overtime and observe the occurrence of the outcome. Cross-sectional study does not have this advantage, and even case-control study does not really distinguish exposure from outcome.

1.3.5 *Experimental Study*

This study must involve experimentation or intervention. Experimental study can be done on animal, patients or even community. Experimental study is best done with a control group, which is the group of subject without any intervention applied. There are also many studies with more than one treatment group. For example is when we want to measure the effect of the drug at different dosages.

Another important feature of an experimental study or trial is the specific characteristic of subjects enrolled as samples. Usually the **selection criteria**[4] are strict to ensure only subjects with specific conditions will be experimented. If clinicians are interested to test new lipid lowering agents, the subject should be those with dyslipidaemia and not simply any patient. All other variables that might influence the effect should be the same between groups. The age, distribution of male and female; and severity of illness should be the same. The subjects are then *randomised* into treatment and control groups. In this example, the control can be patients given usual or established drug, and the treatment group is given the newer drug. If we want to study the dose-response relationship, treatment groups must be divided based on different dosage of the newer drug (Fig. 1.8).

1.4 Sampling Terms

Before we can start selecting the study subjects, we should plan the sampling strategy. It can be done by specifying these five terms:

1. Target population
2. Study population

[4]Selection criteria can be specified as inclusion or exclusion criteria. Those statement suitable as inclusion is written under inclusion criteria, and those suitable as exclusion are listed under exclusion criteria. We should not write, for example, male as one of the inclusion criteria and female as the exclusion because once we stated male as the inclusion criteria, it is automatically known that female should not be included (or should be excluded) in the study.

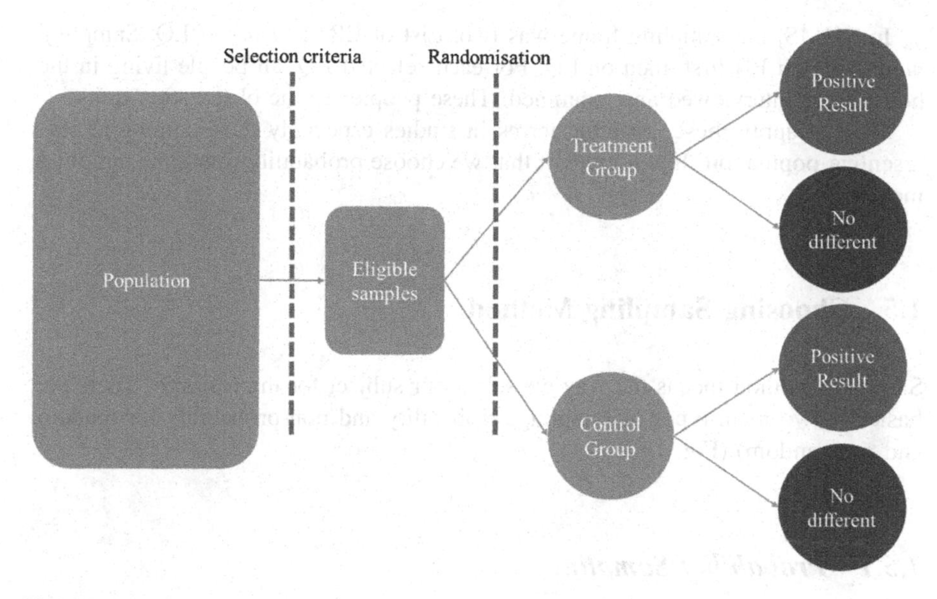

Fig. 1.8 Experimental study design

3. Sampling frame
4. Sampling unit
5. Observation unit

Target population is the population where we will infer the results of the research. Study population is the subset of target population and it must be able to represent target population. Study population is the population that we can reach. For example in National Health and Morbidity Survey (NHMS) III[5] in 2006, the target is all Malaysian but the study population is the household population. The study, however, did not cover Malaysian in institutional residences like hostels, army camps or correctional centres.

Sampling frame is the list of sampling unit. Sampling unit is the characteristic that is being sample. In NHMS, the sampling units were Enumeration Block (EB) and Living Quarter (LQ).

EB is defined as geographical area which is artificially created to have about 80–120 living quarters. In general, it has boundaries, such as natural boundaries—for example, rivers; administrative boundaries—for example, *mukim* or administrative district boundaries; man-made boundaries—for example, roads or railway tracks; imaginary boundaries (straight line) which conjoin places on the map and in some solutions, EBs do not have clear-cut boundaries. EBs may consist of only few localities or villages which are inaccessible by road, for example: Orang Asli settlements in Peninsular Malaysia and rural areas in the interior of Sabah and Sarawak (Department of Statistics Malaysia 2014).

[5]The third 10-yearly national survey on health by Ministry of Health Malaysia.

In NHMS, the sampling frame was two. List of EBs and list of LQ. Sampling were done on EB first, then on LQ. For each selected LQ, all people living in the house were interviewed and examined. These people are the observation units.

We can apply these sampling terms in studies especially those aiming at representing population. It is important that we choose probability (random) sampling method.

1.5 Choosing Sampling Method

Sampling method means the way we select our subject for the research. There are basically two main types of sampling, probability and non-probability (or random and non-random) (Fig. 1.9).

1.5.1 Probability Sampling

Probability sampling means that each sample should have **equal chance** to be selected. If it is truly random, we should not be able to duplicate the technique to get the exact same samples again.

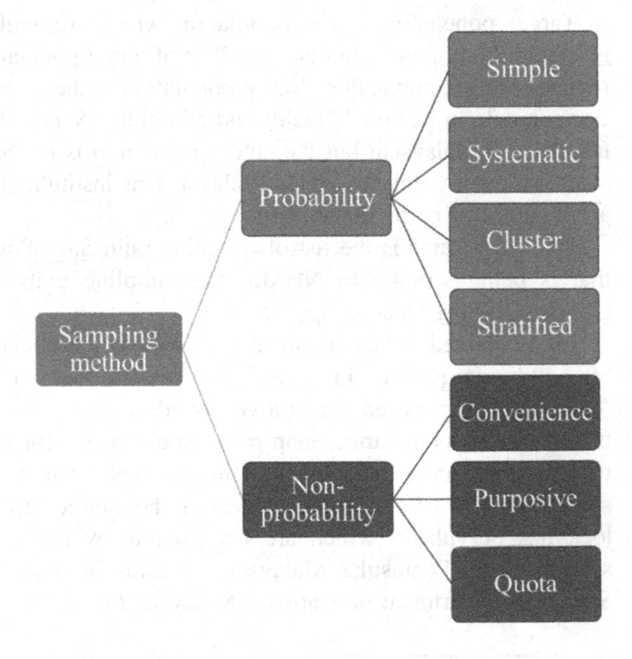

Fig. 1.9 Type of sampling method

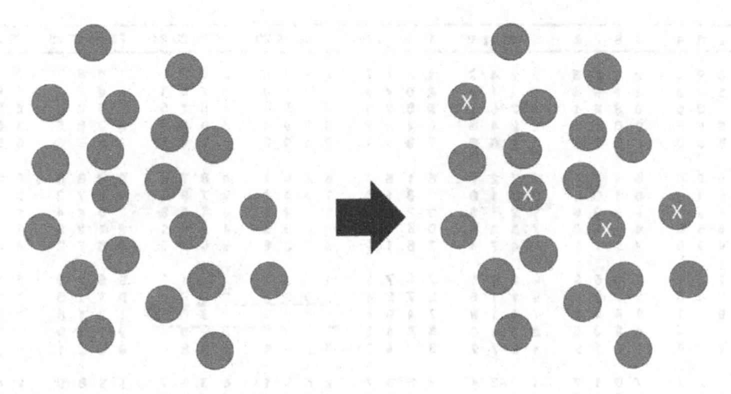

Fig. 1.10 Simple random sampling

1.5.2 Simple Random Sampling

This is the simplest form of sampling and the ideal method. If we have 20 subjects, and we wish to sample only 4 of them (Fig. 1.10), what we can do is draw lots. We write each of their names on a piece of small paper, roll them and put into a bowl. Without looking, randomly draw four of those rolled papers. Alternatively we can use random table (Fig. 1.11). Assign number to the initial 20 subjects, select one number randomly, for example, use a pencil and blindly drop the tip of the pencil onto the paper and choose the nearest number, then choose the subsequent 3 unique numbers. It does not matter which direction you go. The numbers are all random.

For an example, if we plan to select 4 samples from a list of 20 patients; first we sort the name alphabetically (or in any order), then we assign a number from 1 to 20. We dropped the tip of the pencil on to the paper with the random number without looking at it. If the pencil pointed to location near Row 13 and Column 24, the nearest number is 8. Since our population is only 20 names, the number should not exceed 2 digits. So we take number 68. Since we have up to 20 numbers, we choose number 8 instead. Actually all numbers in table are random. So we do not need to repeat the sampling up to 4 times for 4 samples. What we can do is to select all the subsequent numbers instead. We need to decide which direction to move prior to the sampling to avoid bias. Let say we plan to move to the left, so we should select number 68, 73, 65 and 81, and we only use number 8, 3, 5 and 1.

Remember that the key point is that we should not be able to replicate this process. This is crucial when we use software to calculate random number. Software that is able to repeat exactly the same order is not actually random enough.

1.5.3 Systematic Random Sampling

The main difference between simple and systematic random sampling is the frequency of 'random' sampling process. In simple random sampling above, to select

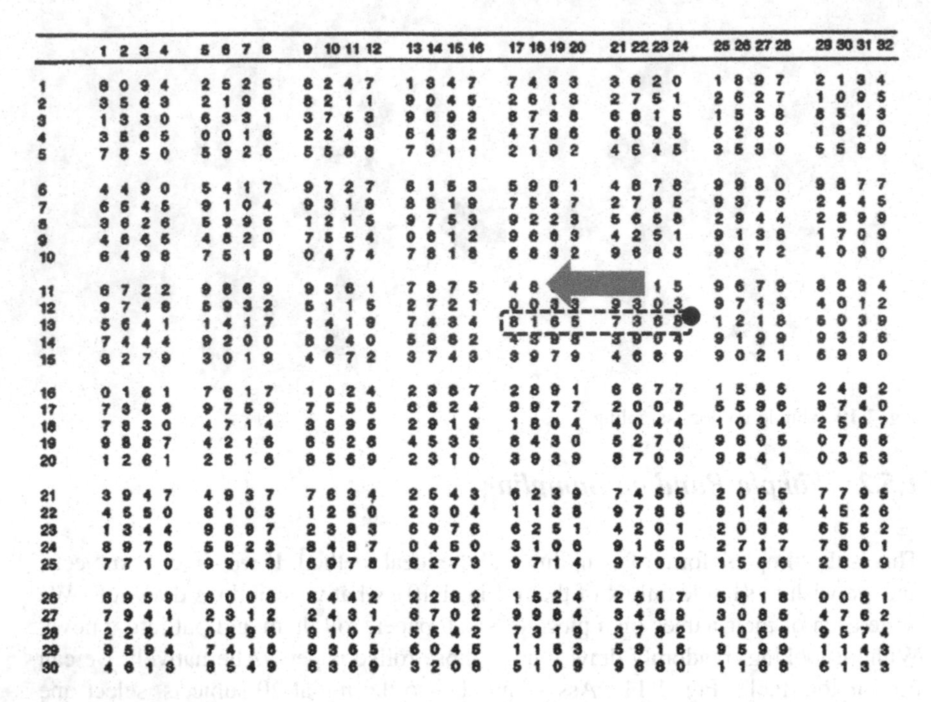

	1 2 3 4	5 6 7 8	9 10 11 12	13 14 15 16	17 18 19 20	21 22 23 24	25 26 27 28	29 30 31 32
1	8 0 9 4	2 5 2 5	8 2 4 7	1 3 4 7	7 4 3 3	3 6 2 0	1 8 9 7	2 1 3 4
2	3 5 6 3	2 1 9 8	8 2 1 1	9 0 4 5	2 6 1 8	2 7 5 1	2 6 2 7	1 0 9 5
3	1 3 3 0	6 3 3 1	3 7 5 3	9 8 9 3	8 7 3 8	6 8 1 5	1 5 3 8	8 5 4 3
4	3 5 6 5	0 0 1 6	2 2 4 3	6 4 3 2	4 7 9 6	6 0 9 5	5 2 8 3	1 6 2 0
5	7 8 5 0	5 9 2 5	5 5 8 8	7 3 1 1	2 1 9 2	4 5 4 5	3 5 3 0	5 5 8 9
6	4 4 9 0	5 4 1 7	9 7 2 7	6 1 5 3	5 9 0 1	4 8 7 8	9 9 8 0	9 8 7 7
7	6 5 4 5	9 1 0 4	9 3 1 8	8 8 1 9	7 5 3 7	2 7 8 5	9 3 7 3	2 4 4 5
8	3 6 2 6	5 9 9 5	1 2 1 5	9 7 5 3	9 2 2 3	5 6 5 8	2 9 4 4	2 8 9 9
9	4 6 6 5	4 8 2 0	7 5 5 4	0 6 1 2	9 6 8 3	4 2 5 1	9 1 3 8	1 7 0 9
10	6 4 9 8	7 5 1 9	0 4 7 4	7 8 1 8	6 8 3 2	9 6 8 3	9 8 7 2	4 0 9 0
11	6 7 2 2	9 8 6 9	9 3 6 1	7 8 7 5	4 8 [illegible]	[illegible] 1 5	9 6 7 9	8 8 3 4
12	9 7 4 8	5 9 3 2	5 1 1 5	2 7 2 1	0 0 3 3	9 3 0 3	9 7 1 3	4 0 1 2
13	5 6 4 1	1 4 1 7	1 4 1 9	7 4 3 4	8 1 6 5	7 3 6 8	1 2 1 8	5 0 3 9
14	7 4 4 4	9 2 0 0	8 8 4 0	5 8 8 2	4 5 9 8	3 9 0 4	9 1 9 9	9 3 3 6
15	8 2 7 9	3 0 1 9	4 6 7 2	3 7 4 3	3 9 7 9	4 6 8 9	9 0 2 1	6 9 9 0
16	0 1 6 1	7 6 1 7	1 0 2 4	2 3 8 7	2 8 9 1	6 6 7 7	1 5 8 6	2 4 8 2
17	7 3 8 8	9 7 5 9	7 5 5 6	6 6 2 4	9 9 7 7	2 0 0 8	5 5 9 6	9 7 4 0
18	7 8 3 0	4 7 1 4	3 6 9 5	2 9 1 9	1 8 0 4	4 0 4 4	1 0 3 4	2 5 9 7
19	9 8 8 7	4 2 1 6	6 5 2 6	4 5 3 5	8 4 3 0	5 2 7 0	9 6 0 5	0 7 6 8
20	1 2 6 1	2 5 1 6	8 5 6 9	2 3 1 0	3 9 3 9	8 7 0 3	9 8 4 1	0 3 5 3
21	3 9 4 7	4 9 3 7	7 6 3 4	2 5 4 3	6 2 3 9	7 4 5 5	2 0 5 6	7 7 9 5
22	4 5 5 0	8 1 0 3	1 2 5 0	2 3 0 4	1 1 3 8	9 7 8 8	9 1 4 4	4 5 2 6
23	1 3 4 4	9 6 9 7	2 3 8 3	6 9 7 6	6 2 5 1	4 2 0 1	2 0 3 8	6 5 5 2
24	8 9 7 6	5 8 2 3	8 4 8 7	0 4 5 0	3 1 0 6	9 1 6 6	2 7 1 7	7 6 0 1
25	7 7 1 0	9 9 4 3	6 9 7 8	8 2 7 3	9 7 1 4	9 7 0 0	1 5 6 6	2 8 8 9
26	6 9 5 9	6 0 0 8	8 4 4 2	2 2 8 2	1 5 2 4	2 6 1 7	5 8 1 8	0 0 8 1
27	7 9 4 1	2 3 1 2	2 4 3 1	6 7 0 2	9 9 8 4	3 4 6 9	3 0 8 6	4 7 6 2
28	2 2 8 4	0 8 9 8	9 1 0 7	5 6 4 2	7 3 1 9	3 7 8 2	1 0 6 8	9 5 7 4
29	9 5 9 4	7 4 1 6	9 3 6 5	6 0 4 5	1 1 8 3	5 9 1 6	9 5 9 9	1 1 4 3
30	4 6 1 3	8 5 4 9	6 3 6 9	3 2 0 8	5 1 0 9	9 6 8 0	1 1 6 8	6 1 3 3

Fig. 1.11 Example of a random number table (Taken from Hill AB (1977) A Short Textbook of Medical Statistics. J. B. Lippincott Company, (Hill 1977))

4 samples out of 20 subjects, the 'random' sampling has to be done 4 times (unless we use random table). For systematic random sampling, you may need only once.

The easiest way is, if we wish to sample 4 from 20 subjects, *sort* the subject first, maybe using their names. Then divide the subjects into 4 groups (because we want 4 subjects). In this example, we will have 5 subjects per group. Then randomly select one number from number 1 to 5. If number 3 is selected, then take those in number 3 position **from each group** (Fig. 1.12).

1.5.4 Cluster Random Sampling

In cluster random sampling subjects were distributed, ideally in homogenous groups that we called cluster. If we wish to represent a state, and the state have 4 relatively equal districts, in term of number, demographic characteristics; then depending on sample size required, for example, if we need to select only 1 district, we can simply select 1 out of 4 available district randomly. That one district selected shall represent the entire state. If we have decided to sample one district, we can proceed to sample the entire people in that. We may sample just some of them for logistic reason. It would be cost effective to concentrate on one district rather than going around getting samples from all 4 districts (Fig. 1.13).

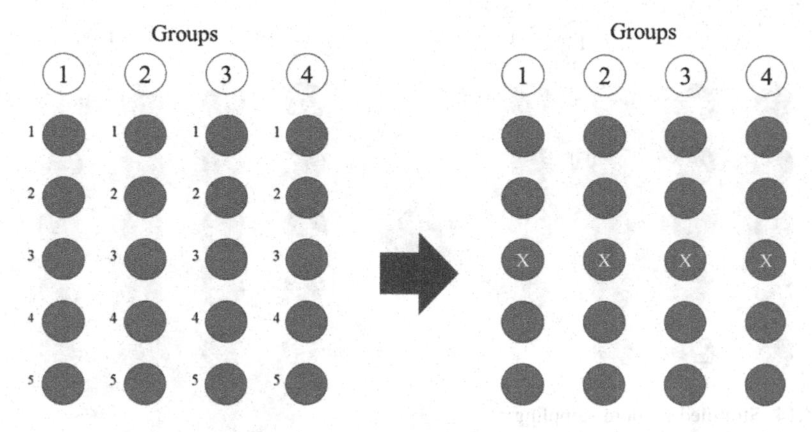

Fig. 1.12 Systematic random sampling

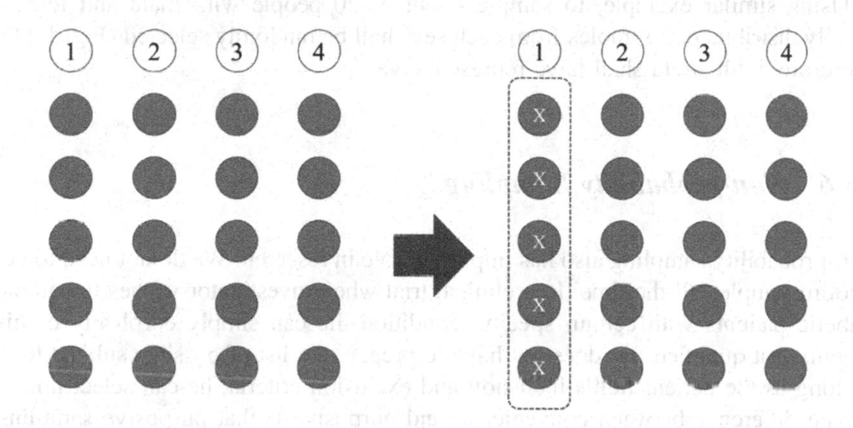

Fig. 1.13 Cluster sampling

However, if the clusters are not exactly homogenous, which is pretty common, this technique will introduce bias in the measurement of variance. This is known as *design effect* (Killip et al. 2004) and need to be accounted for in sample size calculation and analysis.

1.5.5 Stratified Random Sampling

Like cluster random sampling, in stratified random sampling, subjects will be divided in groups, but this time, it is called ***strata***. The difference is, in stratified random sampling, ***all*** strata must be selected, and the strata are determined based on certain characteristics such as sex, age groups and location.

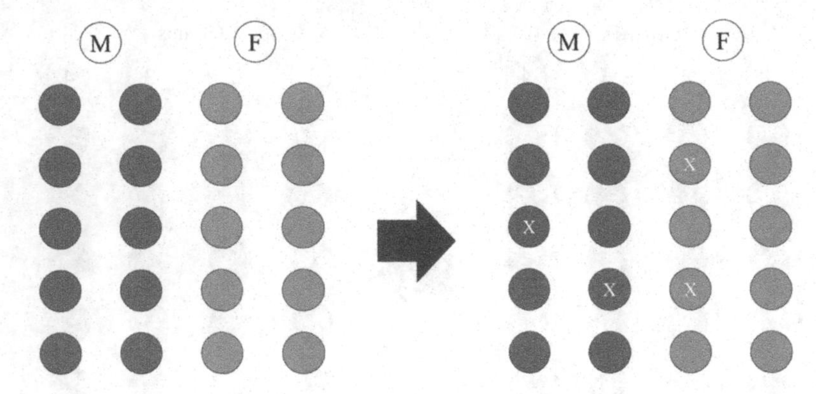

Fig. 1.14 Stratified random sampling

Using similar example, to sample 4 out of 20 people with male and female equally distributed, 2 samples from each sex shall be randomly selected (Fig. 1.14). Therefore, both strata shall have representative.

1.5.6 Non-probability Sampling

Non-probability sampling also has important role in research. We do not need to get random samples all the time. In a clinical trial when investigator wishes to sample diabetic patients with certain specific condition, he can simply enrol any of his patients that qualified. He does not have to prepare the list of possible subject first. As long as the patient fulfils inclusion and exclusion criteria, he can select him.

The difference between convenience and purposive is that purposive sampling has a list of selection criteria. The patient selected must possess those criteria. Where else those selected haphazardly without any guide or criteria are called convenience sampling. Quota sampling is sampling process that stops immediately when we reached certain number of samples.

1.6 Calculating Sample Size

Sample size is essential in almost all research. It is "almost" and not "must" for all research because there are situations when sample size is not required. If we plan to conduct a novel study or a discovery research, something that is never been done before, the sample size does not really important. First, because there is no information about it, so whatever we discover should be the new thing. Second, because when we discover something really important, even if it comes from one sample, it is still a significant finding. In 1869 it was Paul Langerhans, a medical student who discovered about an area of pancreas that produce juice with unknown function. Such discovery does not require sample size calculation.

However, majority of research do require the calculation of sample size. There are many formula exist and it is beyond this book to cover them all. We shall cover those which are really common.

Sample size depends on our main research objective. We can divide them into studies that trying to *represent population* at large or study that focus in measuring association or *testing hypothesis*. Please take note that sample size is **an estimate**, calculated from **previous study** or from **our expectation**.

1.6.1 Sample Size for Population-Based Study

For this study, our main aim is to infer whatever finding we obtained to the population. It can represent a district, state or even country. Usually population here referred to population within certain geographical boundaries. Examples include study to measure prevalence of hypertension in a state or district, study to describe characteristics of diabetic patients in one country etc.

Factors that determine the sample size are listed in Table 1.2. *Expected outcome* is the researcher's expected value for the main outcome. The value can be estimated from previous studies done elsewhere or if not available, the researcher needs to estimate the expected value for the outcome.

Desired precision is the variation from this expected outcome. If we would like to measure prevalence of hypertension in a district, from literatures we found out that the national level was 35 % and we believe the prevalence of hypertension in the study area should be around that value, we can expect that 35 % is the outcome of our study. However, we can only guess, hence the actual result may vary. We need to provide best estimated **variation**. Again we need to refer back to some previous researches done. If based on the literatures, the results were between 30 and 40 %, then we can say that our precision for the estimate is about 5 % (from 35 %). The more precise our expectation is (i.e. the smaller the variation expected), the bigger will be the sample size required. This is pretty similar to the analogy of hitting bull's eye in archery. The smaller the target board, the more precise the shot has to be. For the same archer, more arrows have to be released to hit a smaller target board compared to when using bigger board. In population-based research if the population is very heterogeneous (in term of socio-demographic characteristics

Table 1.2 Factors that affect sample size calculation

1.	Estimate of expected outcome
2.	Desired precision level (margin of error)
3.	Design effect (*Deff*)
4.	Number of strata
5.	Estimated response rate

for example), the less likely for us to obtain precise result. We should expect higher variation. Hence, more sample required to achieve precise estimates.

Design effect (*Deff*) is first mentioned by Kish in 1965 (Kish 1965). It is basically considering the effect of sampling design in research. Anything that is not using simple random sampling as sampling method need to be adjusted and the sample size has to take this into consideration. Those with high-design effect requires higher sample size.

All research that try to represent population must consider all these information in the sample size calculation.

The choice of sample size calculation depends on the *level of measurement*[6] of the main outcome. For example, in the obesity study, usually the main outcome i.e. obese, is measured in categorical form as obese or not obese (dichotomous). Obesity can also be measured using body fat percent which is in numeric.

1.6.2 Sample Size for a Single Proportion

Single proportion here means study that the main objective is to measure the proportion. For an example, a study to measure the prevalence of hypertension as mentioned above. The *suggested*[7] formulae is:

$$n = \frac{\left(z_{\frac{\alpha}{2}}\right)^2 p(1-p)}{d^2},$$

where, p is the expected outcome, d is the precision required and z is the value (using z distribution) for confidence at α confidence level.[8] Usually the α is set to 0.05 and therefore z value at $\frac{0.05}{2}$ is 1.96.

So using the same hypothetical example, expecting the prevalence of hypertension of 35 % with precision of 5 % using α of 0.05, the sample size, n is:

$$n = \frac{1.96^2 \times 0.35(1 - 0.35)}{0.05^2} = 349.6$$

---

[6]Level of measurements include nominal (dichotomous), ordinal and continuous. Please refer to Sect. 1.7.2.

[7]All the formula mentioned are suggested formula rather than ideal ones. The list of formula available to calculate sample size are exhaustive. The formulae are also simplified for most research. Detail considerations, for example, testing difference versus equality, are not discussed here.

[8]Confidence level is the degree of confident that the sample selected represents the true value (of the population parameter).

However, this is correct if the sampling is planned using simple random sampling. If not, the sample size should take account for *Deff*. *Deff* is also an estimate that is based on previous research. The common value used is 1.5. Therefore if *Deff* is 1.5, the sample size is now 349.6 × 1.5 = 524.4.

That is still not the final sample size. The next thing to consider is the *response rate*. If we do household survey, there might be some people who refuse to participate. We should anticipate how many will refuse or may not be at home when we visit them. If the non-response rate is 20 %, the sample size need to be increase another 20 %. So now the sample size should be 629.3. If the study planned does not include stratification, this could be the minimum target sample size. However, if the sampling involves stratification, the number of *strata* has to be included in the calculation. In planning for sample size, we should always remember than sample size planned is always an estimate. So figure should be round up to maybe 630.

1.6.3 Sample Size for a Single Mean

For research with continuous measurement for its outcome, for example fasting blood glucose in mmol/L, the suggested formula is:

$$n = \frac{\left(z_{\alpha/2}\right)^2 \sigma^2}{d^2},$$

where, σ is the standard deviation, $z_{\alpha/2}$ is z value at confidence level, $\alpha/2$ (which is 1.96) and d is the precision required.

If we would like to study mean blood glucose with known standard deviation and precision required of 0.5 and 0.1 mmol/L, respectively, at 95 % confidence interval, the minimum required sample size n, is:

$$n = \frac{1.96^2 \times 0.5^2}{0.1^2} = 96.04.$$

Similarly to the previous exercise above, if the design effect is 1.5, non-response rate of 20 % and no stratification involved, the final sample size is 172.9, rounded to 175 subjects.

Looking at the formula we know that in heterogeneous population, i.e. the higher the standard deviation (σ), the higher the sample size; and likewise if the precision (d) required is higher, i.e. the value is lower.

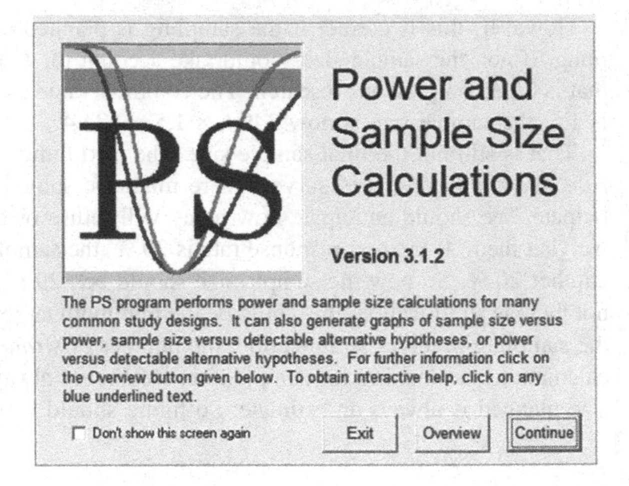

Fig. 1.15 PS: Power and Sample Size Calculation software

1.6.4 Sample Size for Two Proportions

When our aim of a research is to compare values, whether between treatment and control groups, or values pre versus post intervention; we should use formulae that compare the values. The formulae are depending on what statistical test we plan to use and there are many options. The practical approach is using sample size software. I would recommend using PS: Power and Sample Size Calculation (Dupont and Plummer Jr 1990) (Fig. 1.15).

Using the software, if we plan to compare proportion of smoking behaviour between normal subjects and lung cancer patients in a case–control study, we can use *Dichotomous* tab because the variables we wish to compare are dichotomous i.e. smoking or not smoking. If the values are 30 versus 40 % we can enter as presented in Screen 1.1.

m is the ratio of sample size between the two districts which normally we assume the same, hence normally the value is 1. This formula basically using χ^2 test with corrected by Fisher's Exact Test. Prospective was chosen rather than case–control because this is not a case–control study design. Finally when we *Calculate*, as depicted in Screen 1.2, we need around 380 subjects per group. Altogether we need 760 subjects. But do not forget to account for non-response as mentioned previously.

1.6.5 Sample Size for Two Means

If we wish to compare mean blood sugar of between male and female with expected difference of 0.5 mmol/L and estimated of 1 mmol/L *within group standard*

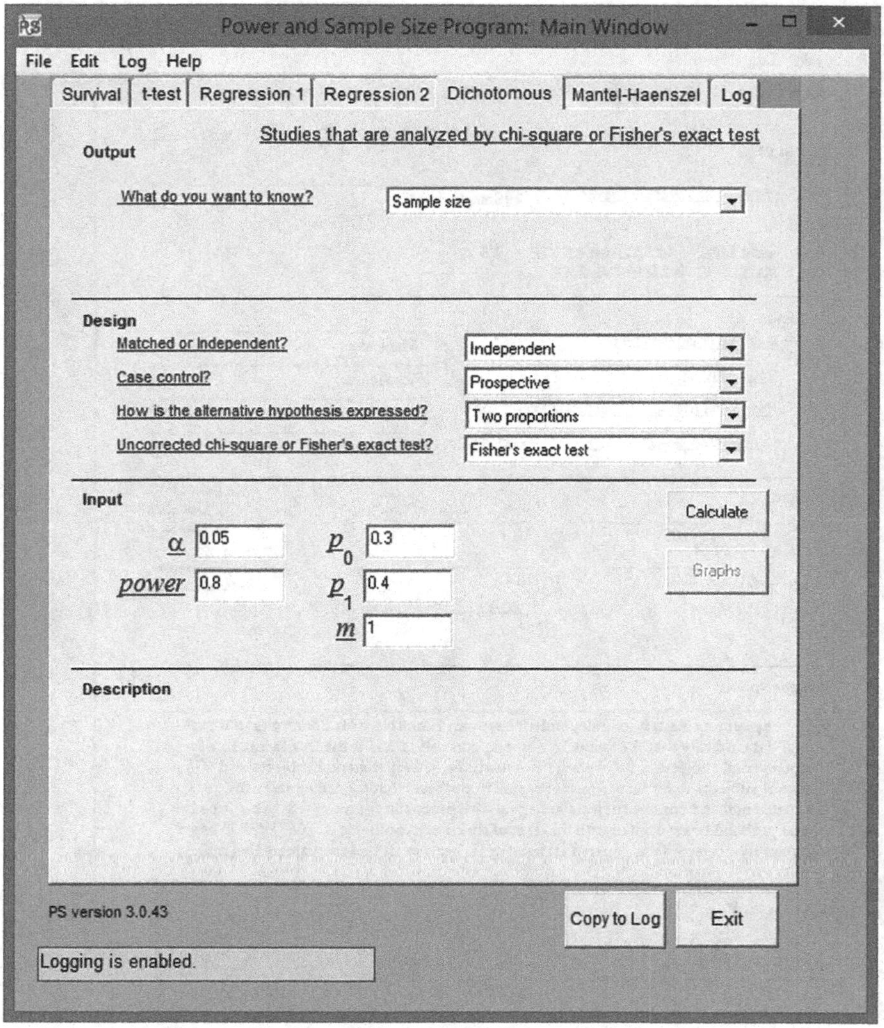

Screen 1.1 Calculate sample size for comparing two proportion using software

deviation,[9] the sample size calculated is 64 per group (Screen 1.3). Altogether you need around 130 subjects. Anticipating 20 % non-response, you may end up with up to 160 total subjects.

---

[9]Within group standard deviation means the standard deviation of that blood sugar for each group. If you have two groups, you may have two different standard deviations, but for sample size calculation we choose the biggest possible value to represent both estimates. The value is your estimation based on previous studies from literature review or from your pilot study.

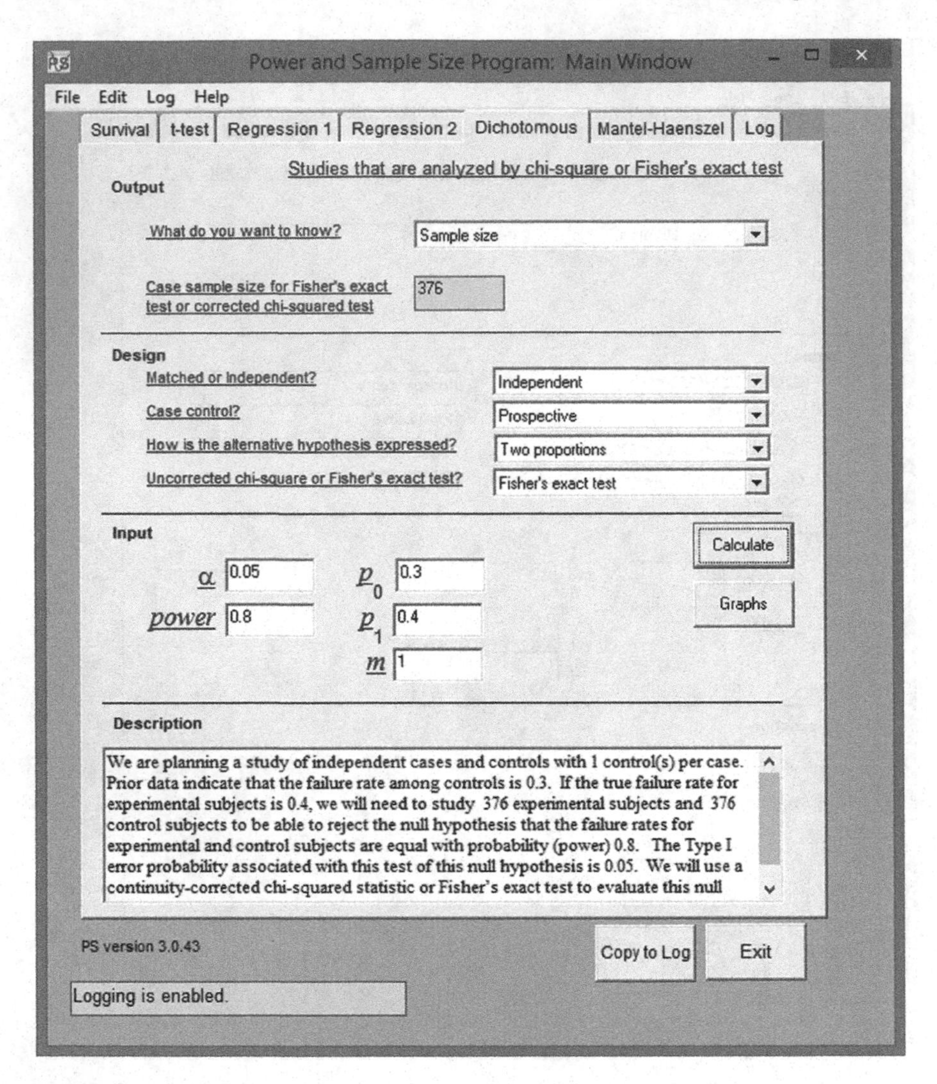

Screen 1.2 The sample size calculated

We chose independent in the *Design* box because mean blood sugar in male is not related to mean blood sugar in female.

If we do a study to compare two blood sugar levels before and after treatment, we should use *Paired* instead because the next level is affected by the previous level. If the values are all the same, this gives smaller sample size (Screen 1.4).

PS: Power and Sample Size Calculation software allows only comparison of two groups. For more advanced sample size calculation, more advanced software is required. Please consult your statistician for that matter.

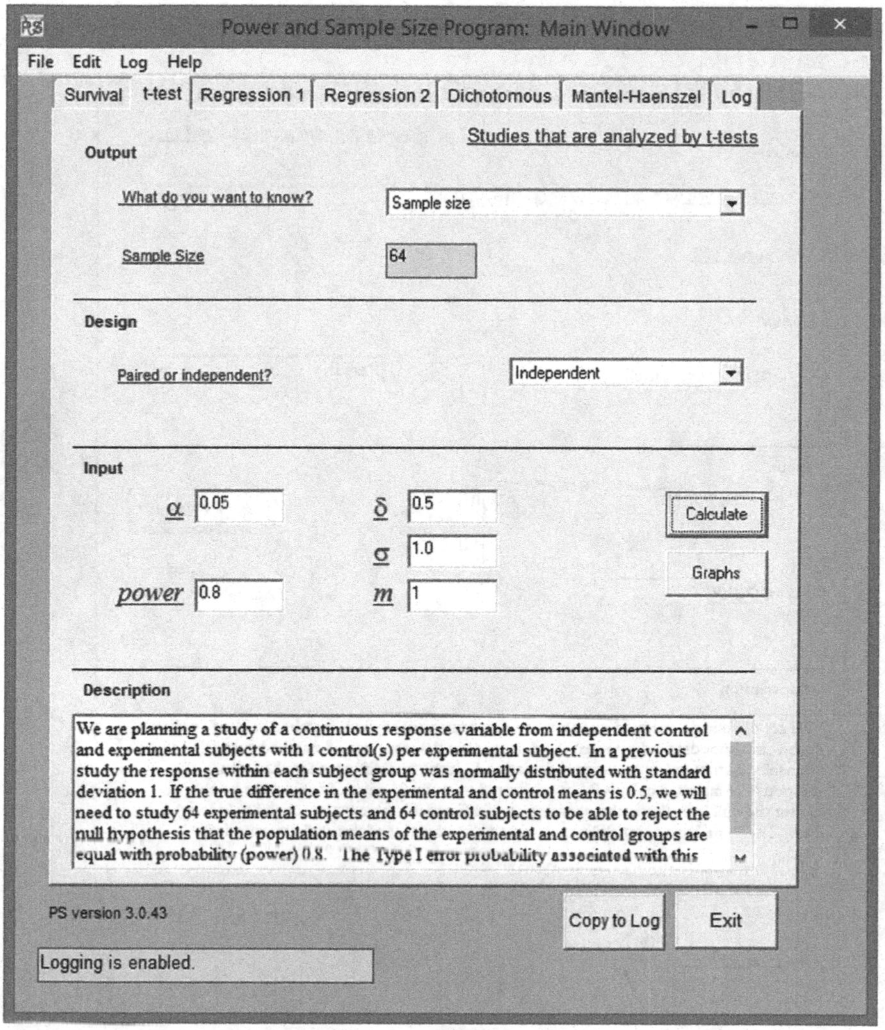

Screen 1.3 Sample size for comparing means using software

1.7 Observations and Measurements

Once we have decided on the design, sampling method and sample size; we should then plan properly on how to collect the data. However, before we can start collecting the data, we should define them properly.

Datum (singular for data), or variable, is characteristics or number that is observed (or measured) and can take any value. Examples are age, gender, salary grade, blood pressure, blood glucose, severity of cancer and success of treatment.

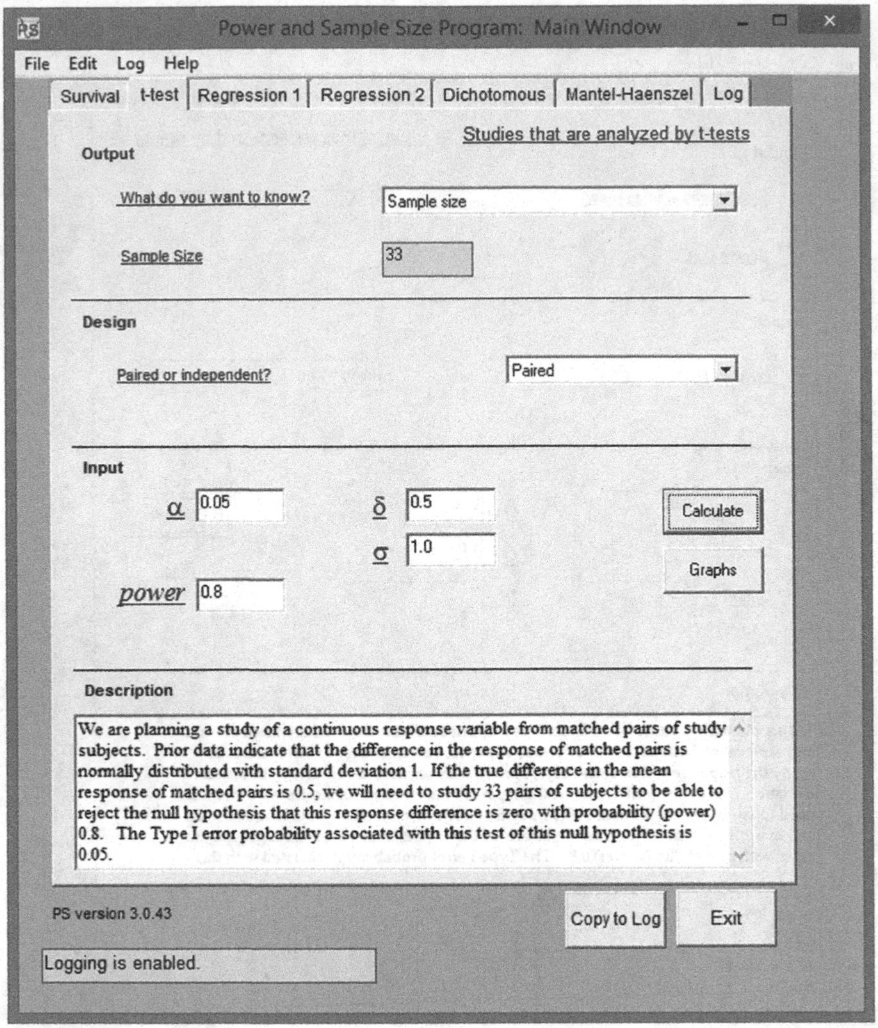

Screen 1.4 Sample size for comparing paired means using software

When we observe a person, he is at certain age with specific gender, receives certain amount of salary for his work every month, practicing certain lifestyle and may have some diseases. And a different person may and most likely have different values.

If we do a study among male smokers, gender is not a variable anymore because we already specified that the samples are all male. So gender is a constant here, and therefore we do not need to collect information on gender.

1.7.1 Role of a Variable

Every variable we wish to measure in a research should have its specific role. We should not collect variable that is not going to fulfil the objective of the research. When *causality* is being investigated, at least a relationship of two variables involved. One variable is considered as the outcome, or dependent variable; whilst another as factor or exposure, or also known as independent variables (Fig. 1.2). As mentioned in previous chapter, it is important to ascertain which variables are dependent and which are independent.

1.7.2 Level of Measurement

Not all variables are measured the same way. Some variables can only be counted and presented in percentage and some when measured can provide more information such as mean, median and mode (Fig. 1.16).

Level of measurements are:

1. *Nominal*—Also known as dummy coding. The variables have different categories which are mutually exclusive but not ordered. It shows qualitative difference between categories. Observations are countable (frequency). We can describe mode but not mean or median. Two values nominal is known as dichotomous. E.g. gender, race.
2. *Ordinal*—Variable that shows rank or order. Distance between ranks is not measurable. We can describe using count, mode and median. Mean is used in many studies but it is inappropriate conceptually. E.g. Cancer stage, Likert scale or pain score.
3. *Interval*—The variable has degree of difference but not ratio. The main characteristic is that it has no absolute zero e.g. temperature. 100 °C is hotter than

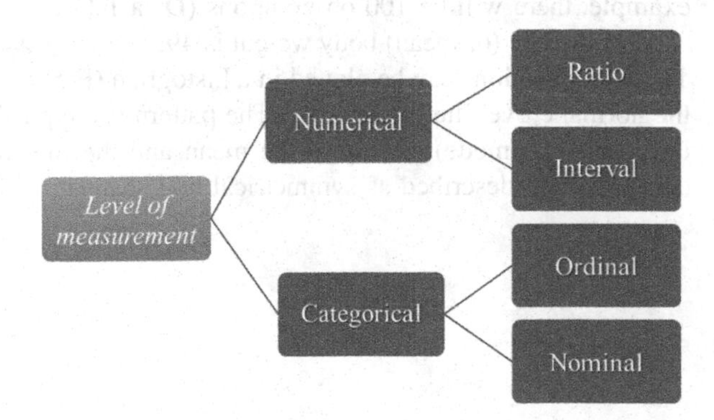

Fig. 1.16 Level of measurement

50 °C but it is not twice hotter. And 0 °C does not mean no temperature. We can measure it by mean, median and mode

4. *Ratio*—The variable has all the properties of interval. It is a measure that shows difference with true zero. We can describe it ratio, mean, median and mode. E.g. Hb, blood sugar, weight etc.

Understanding level of measurement is important because it will affect how we summarise the measurements and what statistics to use. Level of measurement also reflects the 'hierarchy' of measurement. Interval and ratio which belong to numerical measurements provide more information compared to categorical data. However, we do not have to use the same level of measurement when we collect the variables and when we report or analyse them. We need to describe the variables properly. For example, we may capture age in years for the current year but for reporting, we may want to categorise it into old and young taking 60 years as the cut-off point. In this case, age should be treated as categorical when we analyse it. Same goes for other variables like BMI, blood glucose and many others.

It is advisable to collect data in its highest level of measurement and if we wish to categorise them, we can do it later. Those variables collected as categorical cannot be transformed back to its numerical form forever. So be careful when choosing type of variable at the point of data collection.

1.7.3 Data Distribution

If the measurement is numerical, the next characteristic to determine is data distribution. We can describe the distribution using central tendency (measurements) and its dispersion. *Central tendency* means that most of the data are observed at the centre of its distribution. *Dispersion* describes how wide the data spread. Alternatively (even better) we can describe data distribution using histogram (Fig. 1.17).

When we measure body weight among 100 random residences of a village for example, there will be 100 observations (Data 1.1).

The average (or mean) body weight is 49.7 kg with standard deviation of 2.0 kg. These observations can be plotted in a histogram (Fig. 1.15). The thick black line is the normal curve fitted to the data. The pattern is a typical normal distribution with one peak (the mode) exactly at the mean and the median value of the data. The curve is often described as symmetrical bell shaped.

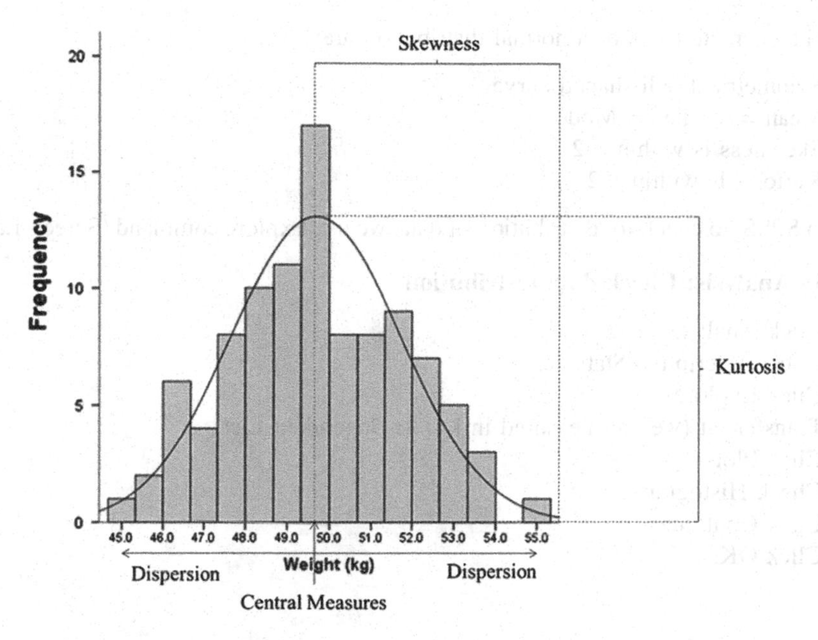

Fig. 1.17 Distribution of body weight (kg)

Data 1.1 Body weights

45.2	47.9	49.3	50.1	51.6
45.7	48.0	49.3	50.1	51.7
45.9	48.1	49.4	50.1	51.7
46.0	48.2	49.4	50.2	51.9
46.1	48.2	49.4	50.3	52.0
46.3	48.2	49.4	50.5	52.1
46.4	48.3	49.4	50.6	52.1
46.5	48.3	49.4	50.7	52.1
46.6	48.3	49.4	50.8	52.2
47.0	48.4	49.5	50.8	52.3
47.2	48.7	49.5	50.8	52.3
47.2	48.7	49.6	50.8	52.7
47.3	48.9	49.6	50.9	52.7
47.5	49.0	49.8	51.0	52.9
47.6	49.0	49.8	51.2	53.0
47.6	49.0	49.9	51.4	53.3
47.7	49.1	49.9	51.4	53.4
47.7	49.1	50.0	51.5	53.4
47.8	49.1	50.0	51.5	53.5
47.9	49.2	50.0	51.5	54.7

The characteristics or a normal distribution are:

1. Symmetrical bell-shaped curve
2. Mean = Median = Mode
3. Skewness is within ± 2
4. Kurtosis is within ± 2

In SPSS, to check for distribution of data, we use Explore command (Screen 1.5).

SPSS Analysis: Check data distribution

1. Click Analyse
2. Click Descriptive Statistics
3. Click Explore
4. Transfer wt (weight measured in kg) to Dependent List
5. Click Plots
6. Check Histogram
7. Click Continue
8. Click OK

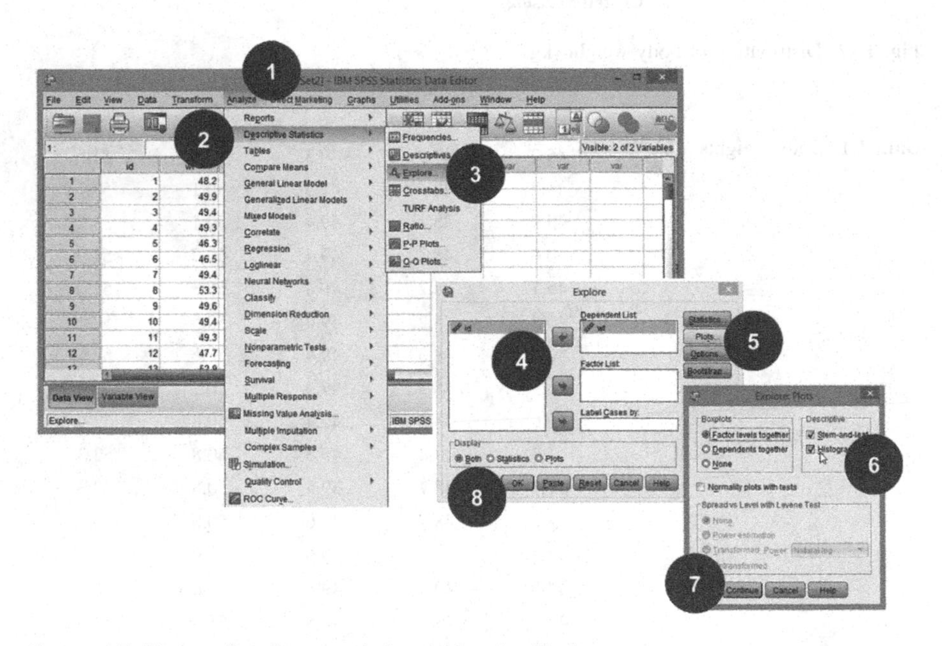

Screen 1.5 How to describe numerical variable using Explore

SPSS Output

Output 1.1 Descriptive statistics for weight

Explore

Case Processing Summary

	Cases					
	Valid		Missing		Total	
	N	Percent	N	Percent	N	Percent
wt	100	100.0%	0	0.0%	100	100.0%

Descriptives

			Statistic	Std. Error
wt	Mean		49.686	.2036
	95% Confidence Interval for Mean	Lower Bound	49.282	
		Upper Bound	50.090	
	5% Trimmed Mean		49.682	
	Median		49.508	
	Variance		4.144	
	Std. Deviation		2.0356	
	Minimum		45.2	
	Maximum		54.7	
	Range		9.5	
	Interquartile Range		3.1	
	Skewness		.049	.241
	Kurtosis		-.492	.478

The Descriptives table describes the weight variable. The mean is 49.7 kg with standard deviation 2.0 kg. The skewness is 0.049 and kurtosis −0.492. These information, together with the Histogram (Fig. 1.17), suggest that the observed body weights are normally distributed.

If the data do not follow these characteristics, we can transform the data. Common transformation includes logarithm, exponentiation or inversion; or we could describe and analyse them differently. This will be discussed in Sect. 2.1.

1.7.4 Preparing Data Dictionary

Data dictionary is a documentation to assist researcher, data enumerator and statistician for their specific task in the research. This information will ensure all terms used in the research are standard and will be interpreted the same way by everyone. All variables required for the research should be identified and then defined carefully. Variables are identified from the conceptual framework. There is

Table 1.3 Suggested information for data dictionary

1	Name	The name normally required in computer such as in data base and statistical analysis. Name can be in one short word e.g. *agecat* for Age Category
2	Label	The name that can appear in table, graph or report
3	Definition	The definition used in the research. It is advisable to include references used. This should also include operational situations e.g. hypertension is diagnosed when the respondent is known to have hypertension either by showing his medical record or the medications he is taking; or systolic blood pressure 140 mmHg or more; and/or diastolic blood pressure of 90 mmHg or more.
4	Instrument used	When relevant, we can describe the instrument used, which includes the brand and the method of calibration if relevant. Credibility of the model used can be referred to established documents.
5	Level of measurement	Should specify either it is nominal, ordinal or continuous
6	Category option and code	If the variable is categorical, the options should be specified e.g. Gender; Male = 1, Female = 2
7	Unit of measurement	If the variable is numerical, we should specify its unit e.g. mmol/L, mg/dL
8	Precision of measurement	How precise the variable is measured e.g. age is measured to the nearest 1-year old. Income is measured to the nearest RM100
9	Data linkage	If this variable is related to other variable, we can specify here e.g. missing value (question on pregnancy) if respondent is Male (question on Gender); or BMI is linked to both variable weight and height.

no one standard template for data dictionary. However, you can always find such document from most major studies.[10] The proposed information required for a data dictionary is presented in Table 1.3.

1.7.5 Validity and Reliability of Research Instrument

To collect or measure the variables in research, we use variety of instruments. We may ask certain questions and the response from the study samples are considered as the value for that variable. Examples of such questions are age, smoking habit, previous history of illness or certain daily routines like exercise. We also use apparatus or machine to help our measurement. For example, we use weighing scale to measure body weight, sphygmomanometer for blood pressure, blood analyser for

[10]For example in NHANES study, their data dictionary is available at http://www.cdc.gov/nchs/data_access/data_linkage/mortality/restricted_use_linked_mortality.htm. Example of data dictionary for Avon Logitudinal Study for Parents and Children, University of Bristol, UK at http://www.bris.ac.uk/alspac/researchers/data-access/data-dictionary/.

blood sugar and even imaging devices such as x-ray machines to assess fracture. These research instrument used, whether the questionnaires or the devices have to be both valid and reliable.

Valid instrument able to measure the actual or the true value. For instance if sphygmomanometer shows blood pressure of 120/80 mmHg, then the blood pressure should be 120/80 mmHg. However, if the device is faulty, or **poor technique** was applied, then it might shows higher or lower than the true value. If the body fat is 30 %, the body fat analyser should read 30 %, not 15 %. The device might be working well but when proper procedure not adhered to during the measurement process e.g. patient was wearing gold bracelet (that increase the conduction), this will impair the proper measurement. When we ask patient's occupation because we believe the occupation might relate to the outcome we are studying, we should specify the **duration**. For example, *"Since the last 12 months, what is or are your occupation?"* If we ask *current occupation*, he might just started doing that job yesterday and that occupation is definitely not able to affect the outcome yet.

Reliable instrument able to produce the same result **repeatedly**. If we measure the blood pressure twice, the readings should be about the same. If the readings keep on changing every minute, something must be wrong with the device.

To measure behavioural variables or anything subjective such as trying to quantify stress, happiness, attitude and awareness; we may need to ask more than one question to get the answer. This involves tedious validation process including identification of content, construct and confirmation of the questionnaire. It is beyond of this book to discuss on how to conduct a validation study.

Validating apparatus or devices is relatively easier. We must make sure the same instrument used throughout the research. The instrument should have documented validity and reliability reports, usually done by the manufacturer, and it is acceptable as **research standard** by the authorities of that area. We must adhere to the **correct procedure** when using the device including proper preparation and positioning of the subjects. For example, when measuring fasting blood sugar, we must make sure the subjects fast accordingly. No point having great and standard blood analyser when the patient is not fasting properly. What we get is random blood sugar and not fasting blood sugar. The instrument must also be **calibrated** according to the schedule. All these procedure should be well documented in the research report.

Valid instrument must be reliable too. We cannot consider the instrument to be valid if it is not reliable. But there are reliable instruments that are not valid i.e. they give same one wrong value repeatedly. For example is a poorly calibrated weighing scale. If it is not done properly, it may weigh higher and lower persistently.

The most common analogy used to explain validity and reliability is the precision of an athlete in archery. The objective is to get the highest possible points by hitting the X ring (the centre) for the full 10 points all the time. If he is very good, he will hit the centre all the time. Able to hit the centre is valid and doing that all the

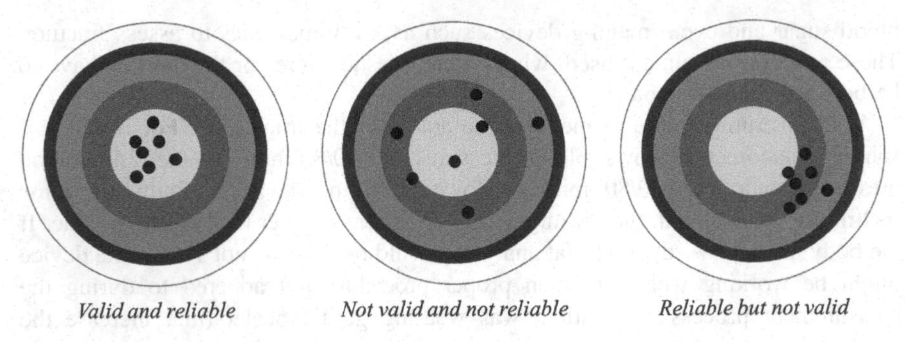

Fig. 1.18 Analogy for validity and reliability

time is reliable. If he hits the centre few times and misses many times, then he is not considered as a good athlete. The arrow may hit the centre by chance and not because he is good (not valid and not reliable). If he is a good archer but failed to adjust the bow properly or he has a problem seeing the board clearly, he may hit the same spot all the time, but the spot is not the centre (Fig. 1.18).

1.8 Data Quality Control

We have *measured* the data properly but we must also make sure they are *recorded* correctly too. Regardless whether we opted for paper-based or electronic-based data entry, there must always be proper quality check at all level.

To ensure data are entered properly into the form, we can assign field supervisor. Ideally he should check all the data but checking certain portion of the entries randomly is also acceptable and more feasible. If a lot of errors identified, the enumerators (data collector) shall be advised and all his records must be scrutinised.

It would be easier if we use electronic data entry. We could design the record form to have certain validation rules. In Malaysia, the identification number (MyKad) can tell us about the age and gender. Assuming the national ID is correct, we can verify respondents' age and gender. We can also set limit to certain variable. For example, we could assign warning when data enumerator enters respondent's age beyond 100-year old as not many people can live beyond that number. The system can ask enumerator to confirm his entry because he might has typed it wrongly. It is also easier to enforce *skip questions* using electronic device. Skip questions is like asking *first day of the last menstrual period* (LMP) for female respondents. Male respondents do not need to answer the question. They can skip it. However, electronic devices require good battery and maybe internet access. There might not be electricity or internet access in the study area, so please study the practicality of using technology for our study area.

More often we collect data on the field using paper-based questionnaire and enter them into the computer elsewhere at later time. To ensure the quality, we could adopt double data entry technique. In this technique, the data in one questionnaire form are entered twice by two different persons. The system should be able to identify data which are entered differently. If occurred, the third person will need to rectify it and enter the correct value.

At the data analysis stage, we can run descriptive statistics to check data range and frequency for categorical variables.

1.9 Plan for Statistical Analysis

A good research must have a complete statistical analysis planned before data collection starts. The plan should explain how we would analyse based on the research objective. Statistical analysis involves both descriptive and analytical statistics. We should describe how we would want to summarise important variables and then we may proceed with more detail analyses including bivariable or even multivariable analyses. The product of a good statistical plan is dummy table. We use the word 'table' here but it could be in the form of figure, graph or even text. Dummy table is basically our expected presentation of the results of the analysis based on our objectives. An example of a dummy table is given in Fig. 1.19.

Objective

To compare blood glucose level between gender

Variables involved

Variable label	*Working definition (linkage data)*	*Status*	*Variable name*	*Level of measurement*	*Category label (if relevant)*	*Variable Unit*	*Precision of measurement*	*Missing value*
Blood glucose	As measured	Dependent	glu	Interval		mmol/L	0.1	999
Gender	As reported	Independent	sex	Nominal	1 = Male, 2 = Female			None

Statistical analysis

1. Check normality of *glu*
2. If *glu* Normal, run Independent sample t-test; if *glu* not Normal, run Mann-Whitney U-Test
3. Significance level = 0.05

Dummy table

	Mean (SD)	*Statistics*	*df*	*P*
Male	nn.n (n.n)	n.nnn	nn	0.nnn
Female	nn.n (n.n)			

SD = Standard deviation

Fig. 1.19 Example of a dummy table

1.10 Critical Information in Research Proposal

In summary, the critical part in planning a research are:

1. Good summary of literature search represented as a ***conceptual framework***
2. SMART-ly phrased ***objectives***
3. Complete and detail ***data dictionary***
4. Clear ***dummy table***

Anyone who is able to provide these four information in their research proposal should face only little problem when doing their research.

Chapter 2
Analysing Research Data

Abstract Data analysis can be divided into two: descriptive and analytical. In descriptive statistics, the main objective is to summarise the variables concerned, usually individually. Analytical statistics the aim is to describe the relationship between two variables or more.

Keywords Descriptive · Analytical · Hypothesis testing · Inferential statistics · Causal · SPSS

Generally, the analysis consists of two parts, descriptive statistics and analytical statistics.

2.1 Descriptive Statistics

The first thing to do before we analyse the data is to describe the variables. When we are studying hypertension in one population, we should first describe the population. We can describe the distribution of age, gender, race, education and income level. We should include the spread, or the precision of the estimates, such as the standard deviation, standard error or confidence interval.

The estimates used to describe a variable depend on the **level of its measurement** (Fig. 2.1). For categorical measures, *frequency* or count with *percentage* should suffice. When we describe distribution of gender, which is a nominal measurement, we could describe the number of male and its percentage over total number. Usually in a variable with two categories data like this, describing one category is enough because the other will complement the value. We do not need to describe frequency and percentage for female.

For numerical measures, it will depend on the **distribution**. If it is a normal distribution, we could use *mean* and its dispersion values such as *standard deviation*. When data are not normally distributed, we should not use mean and its product because **mean is affected by extreme values**. In such situation, *median* is a

J. Ab Rahman, *Brief Guidelines for Methods and Statistics in Medical Research*, SpringerBriefs in Statistics,
DOI 10.1007/978-981-287-925-7_2

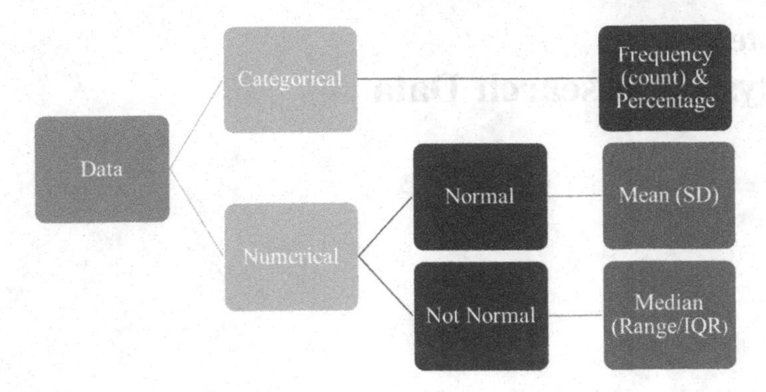

Fig. 2.1 How to describe a variable?

> A study among 150 adults to measure the prevalence of high blood pressure and to describe any factors that may be associated with it. The variables include age (in years), gender, average income per month (RM), smoking status, body mass index (BMI) (kg/m2), fasting blood glucose (mmol/L) and fasting total cholesterol (mmol/L).

Data 2.1 High blood pressure

better alternative. We should not use standard deviation as it is derived from mean. We could use *minimum-maximum* value, *range* or *inter-quartile range*.

To illustrate the points, in this chapter we will be using a hypothetical data (Data 2.1) of a study about hypertension among 150 adults.

2.1.1 Describe Numerical Data

For such study, normally the first thing to do is to describe the demographic characteristics of the study samples. Let us start by analysing the **age** distribution.

SPSS Analysis: Describe numerical data

1. Click Analyze
2. Click Descriptive Statistics
3. Click Explore
4. Move age to Dependent List box
5. Click Plots
6. Check Histogram
7. Click Continue
8. Click OK

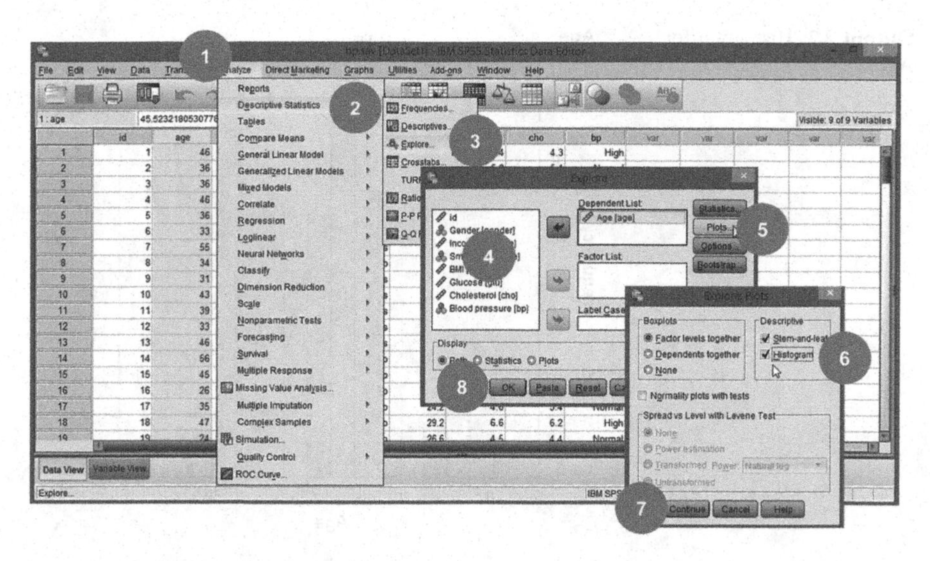

Screen 2.1 How to describe numerical variable using Explore

SPSS Output

The results here show that the mean (SD) is 37.6 (7.6) years, and median (IQR) is 37.5 (10) years, ranging from 18 to 56 years old. Skewness and kurtosis are −0.254 and −0.198, respectively.

Output 2.1 Descriptive statistics of Age

Explore

Case Processing Summary

	Cases					
	Valid		Missing		Total	
	N	Percent	N	Percent	N	Percent
Age	150	100.0%	0	0.0%	150	100.0%

Descriptives

			Statistic	Std. Error
Age	Mean		37.61	.624
	95% Confidence Interval for Mean	Lower Bound	36.38	
		Upper Bound	38.84	
	5% Trimmed Mean		37.74	
	Median		37.48	
	Variance		58.384	
	Std. Deviation		7.641	
	Minimum		18	
	Maximum		56	
	Range		38	
	Interquartile Range		10	
	Skewness		-.254	.198
	Kurtosis		-.198	.394

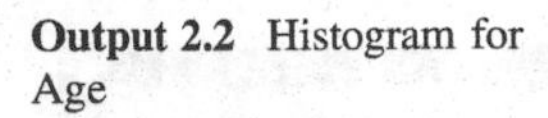

Output 2.2 Histogram for Age

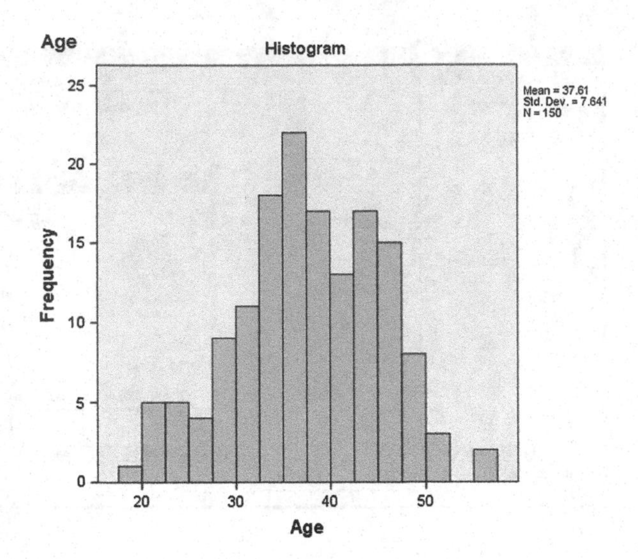

Looking at the histogram above, we might not be able to appreciate its distribution. What we can do is to fit a distribution curve on it.

SPSS Analysis: Fitting normal curve

1. At the output window, double click on the graph to open up Chart Editor
2. Check Show Distribution Curve
3. Close the Properties window (You can skip this step)
4. Close Chart editor

SPSS Output

The distribution curve (Output 2.3) is a symmetrical bell-shaped, hence further strengthen our assumption that age is normally distributed. Therefore, the age should be described using mean and standard deviation.

If you run Explore for glucose, you will realise that glucose is not normally distributed (Output 2.4). The mean is 5.568 mmol/L, the median is 5.218 mmol/L and the histogram with distribution curve (Output 2.5) obviously shows that glucose is skewed to the left (positive skewness, 1.62) and the kurtosis is 3.4. Therefore, to describe glucose, we should use its median and IQR rather than mean and SD.

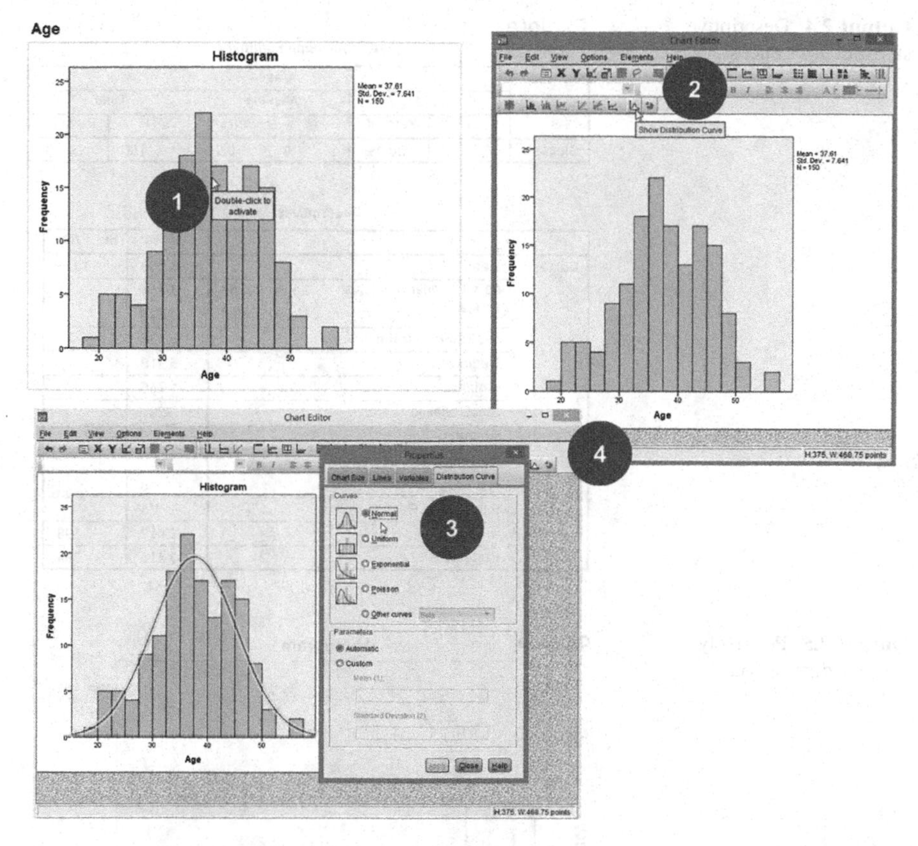

Screen 2.2 How to add Normal curve

Output 2.3 Histogram of Age with Normal curve

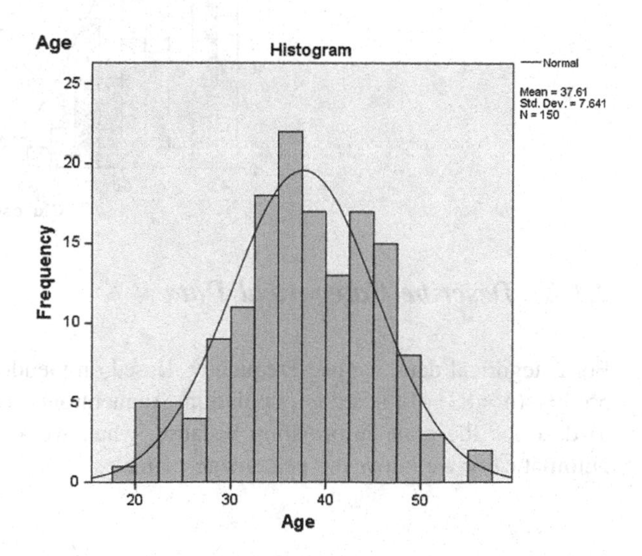

Output 2.4 Descriptive statistics for Glucose

Explore

Case Processing Summary

	Cases					
	Valid		Missing		Total	
	N	Percent	N	Percent	N	Percent
Glucose	150	100.0%	0	0.0%	150	100.0%

Descriptives

			Statistic	Std. Error
Glucose	Mean		5.568	.1085
	95% Confidence Interval for Mean	Lower Bound	5.354	
		Upper Bound	5.783	
	5% Trimmed Mean		5.438	
	Median		5.218	
	Variance		1.765	
	Std. Deviation		1.3287	
	Minimum		4.0	
	Maximum		11.8	
	Range		7.8	
	Interquartile Range		1.5	
	Skewness		1.622	.198
	Kurtosis		3.415	.394

Output 2.5 Positively skewed distribution of Glucose

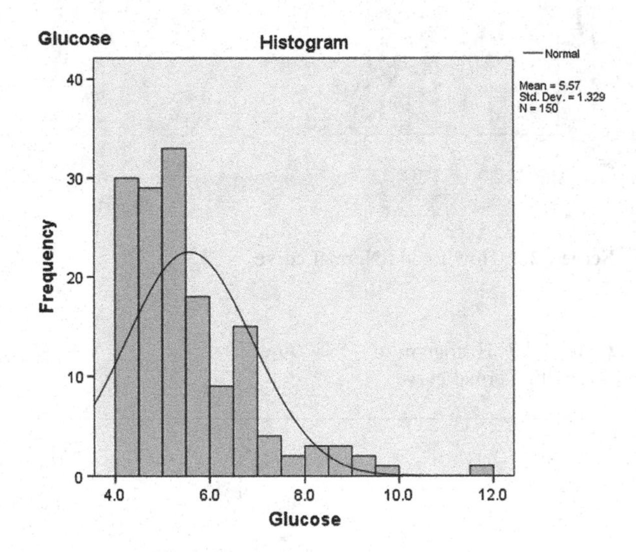

2.1.2 Describe Categorical Data

For categorical data, we use Frequency. Based on Gender table, female constitutes 55.3 % (n = 83) of the study population. As mentioned previously, we do not have to describe the male information because, when we know percentage of female, automatically we know the percentage of male.

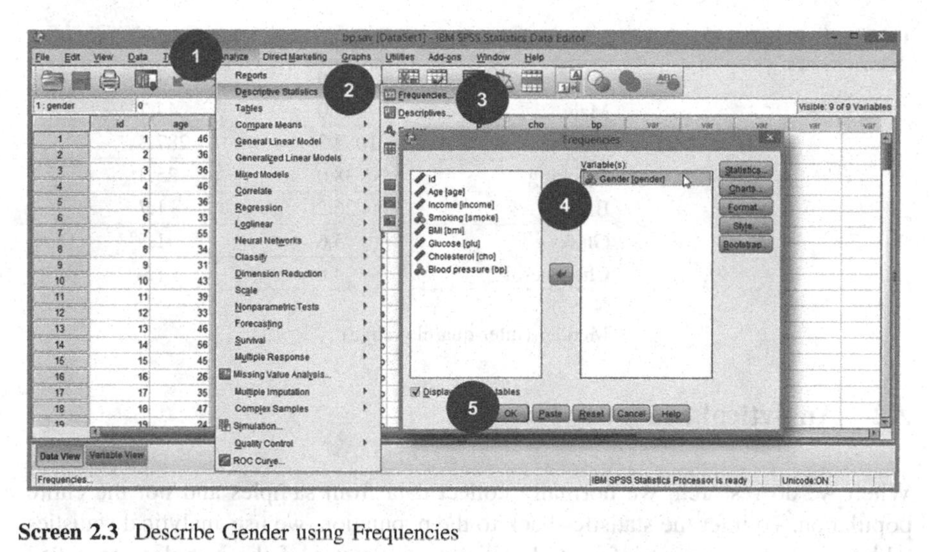

Screen 2.3 Describe Gender using Frequencies

SPSS Analysis: Frequency

1. Click Analyse
2. Click Descriptive Statistics
3. Move gender to Variable(s)
4. Click OK

SPSS Output

We can continue to describe other variables and the suggested presentation of this exercise is presented in Table 2.1.

Output 2.6 Descriptive statistics for Gender

Frequencies

Statistics

Gender

N	Valid	150
	Missing	0

Gender

		Frequency	Percent	Valid Percent	Cumulative Percent
Valid	Female	83	55.3	55.3	55.3
	Male	67	44.7	44.7	100.0
	Total	150	100.0	100.0	

Table 2.1 Baseline characteristics

	Mean	SD
Age	37.6	7.6
Male	67.0	44.7[a]
Income	1082.3	287.3
Smoking	38.0	25.3[a]
BMI	26.2	1.7
Glucose	5.6	1.5[b]
Cholesterol	4.8	1.4

[a]N (%)
[b]Median (Inter-quartile range)

2.2 Analytical Statistics

When we do research, we normally collect data from samples and not the entire population. To infer the statistics back to the population, we use analytical statistics which is also known as inferential statistics. Estimates of the samples are called statistics and those of the population are called parameters. Inferential statistics will measure how close the statistics represent the population. Inferential statistics also means testing theories, or testing hypotheses. If we measure the difference of two estimates derived from a **population**, we do not need any measure to ascertain the precision of the difference because whatever we observed is the actual value. But when we compare statistics from **samples** of the population, the comparison has to be tested for truth.

If we are interested to study blood glucose of all our 100 patients attending our clinic and we managed to sample the whole 100, whatever measurements, such as mean and standard deviation that we calculated, are true and represent the population. However, if we are interested to infer the finding beyond those 100 patients, for example, referring to the diabetic patients in the whole state rather than just the clinic, then the definition of population is no longer limited to those 100 patients. The 100 patients are just a fraction of the entire population of diabetic patients of the state. While the mean and standard deviation may represent the population, we require some form of statistical tests to confirm its validity and precision.

Most of the time in research, this is our aim, inferring the results beyond our samples (Fig. 2.2).

Imagine that we have 35 marble balls (population) with 15 of them are red and the rest are blue in colour (Fig. 2.3). This gives the percentage of red marbles 42.8 % (15/35). If we are to sample only six marbles randomly the percentage of red marbles selected may not be exactly 42.8 % but **around** that value. For example, if in the first sampling we get three reds (out of six marbles selected), the percentage is 50 %. If we put back all the marbles and resample again six marbles, we may get two red marbles (33.3 %); and if we resample the third time, we may get four reds (66.7 %). The **average of those percentages** is 50 %, and even though it is not exactly 42.8 % (the parameter), it is still quite close. The estimates will

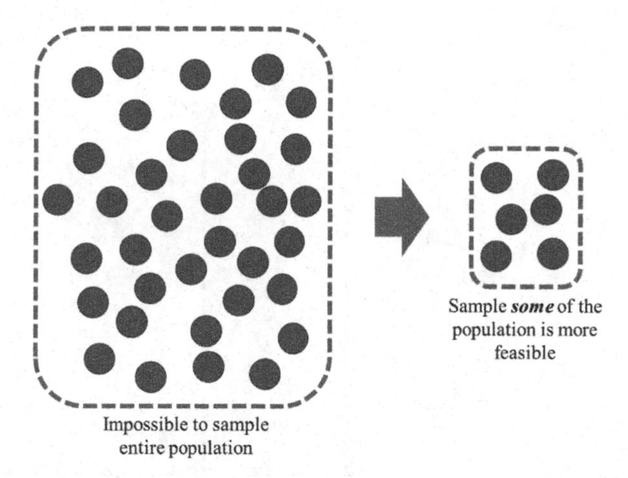

Fig. 2.2 Sampling

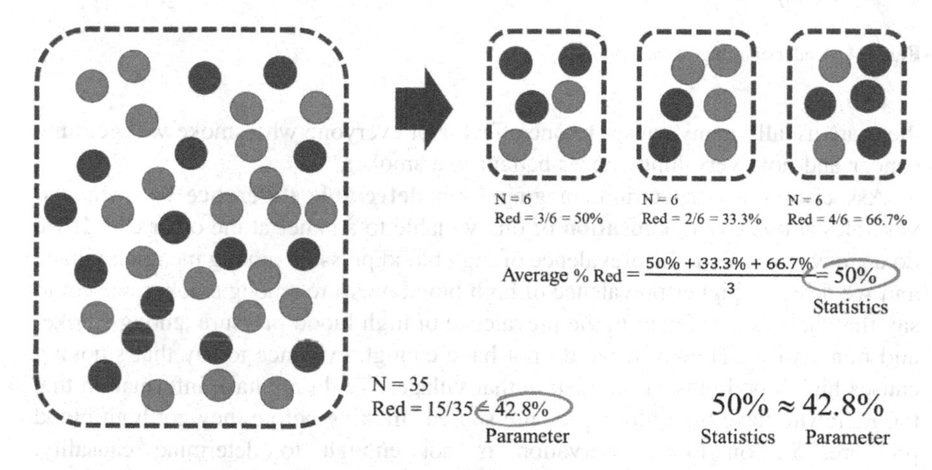

Fig. 2.3 How statistics estimates parameter

become more precise **if more sampling done**. The variation of averages is known as standard error and it is the indication of sampling error. The more the sampling done, the smaller is the sampling error will be, and hence the more precise it represents the population.

2.2.1 Concept in Causal Inference

The ultimate inference we would normally like to make is **causation**. 'A' is causing 'B', such as smoking is causing lung cancer. However, as mentioned in Chap. 1,

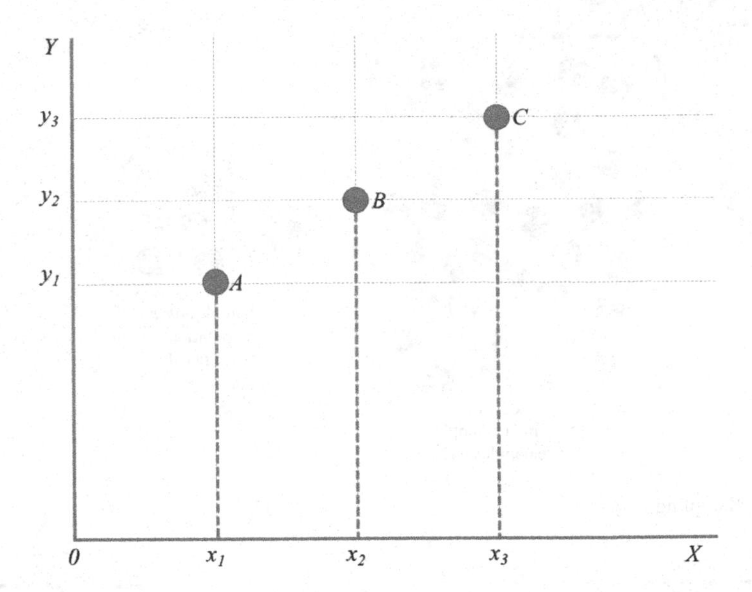

Fig. 2.4 Understanding association

there are usually many causes to one effect. Not everyone who smoke will get lung cancer and not every lung cancer patient is a smoker.

Association is a spectrum, ranging from **detectable difference** between two variables at one end to **causation** of one variable to another at the other end. If we do a study to measure the prevalence of high blood pressure among men in a village and we detected higher prevalence of high blood pressure among smoker, we could say that there is a different in the prevalence of high blood pressure among smoker and non-smoker. However, we do not have enough evidence to say that smoking causes high blood pressure in men in that village. We do not have information that the men who have high blood pressure started smoking before they got high blood pressure. So one-time observation is not enough to determine causality. Furthermore, the difference is detected only true for that instance and might not valid for observation at different times or different populations.

Let us study the association of *X* and *Y* as depicted in Fig. 2.4. There is a difference between observations *A* and *B* which is at x_1 and x_2, respectively. *B* is $y_2 - y_1$ higher than *A*. At this point, we are focusing at the 'difference' and it is not enough to observe anything beyond that. However, when we have information about *C* at x_3, we could now say that not only *C* is higher than *B* by $y_3 - y_2$ but we can also observe a 'trend'. The higher the value of *X*, the higher the value of *Y*. If we have another *x* after x_3, we can even **predict** its *y* value.

So the association between two variables can be from the **difference** of their observations, to the **prediction** of one variable upon another variable. Eventually, when the association is being very persistent we could observe **causation**. Professor Hill outlined eight guidelines to justify causation (Hill 1965):

1. Strength of the association
2. Consistency of the observed association
3. Specificity of the association
4. Temporal relationship of the association
5. The presence of biological gradient or dose-response relationship
6. Coherence with known facts
7. Possible to appeal to experimental evidence

2.2.2 *Hypothesis Testing*

We hypothesise that changes in samples are also happening in the population. But whatever we observed among samples might not occur similarly in the population. Therefore, we need to determine whether the difference or association we observed among samples is also true in the population. We need to test the hypothesis. Let us use the same example about smoking and hypertension. The hypothesis could be that the prevalence of hypertension among smokers is higher than among the non-smokers. If the prevalence of hypertension among smokers is 45 % and non-smokers 40 %, we must decide whether the 5 % difference is true for the population or just occurred coincidently in the sample that we studied. If it is indeed by chance, the value will not be consistent when we repeat it using different sets of samples from the same population.

Hypothesis testing follows the following steps:

1. State the hypothesis
2. Set a criterion to decide
3. Choosing suitable statistical test
4. Make a decision

2.2.3 *State the Hypothesis*

We need to state both null hypothesis (H_o) and alternative hypothesis (H_a). Null hypothesis is a hypothesis of negation. It will always be **a statement to deny the difference.** We may state that there is **no difference** of prevalence between smokers and non-smokers. The alternative hypothesis could be that there is indeed a difference and we do not bother which prevalence is higher (two-tail), or we could also make a more specific alternative hypothesis (one-tail) by saying either prevalence of hypertension among smoker is higher or prevalence among non-smoker is higher. For one-tail hypothesis, we require more evidence to reject its H_o.

	H_o is true	H_o is false
Reject H_o	Type 1 error	Correct decision
Do not reject H_o	Correct decision	Type 2 error

Fig. 2.5 Hypothesis testing

If the P_1 is the prevalence of hypertension among smokers and P_2 as the prevalence of hypertension among non-smokers, H_o is the null hypothesis and H_a as the alternative hypothesis:

$$H_o : P_1 = P_2$$

$$H_a : P_1 - P_2 \neq 0; \quad \text{or} \quad P_1 > P_2; \quad \text{or} \quad P_2 > P_1$$

Our task now is to reject the null hypothesis. Rejecting null hypothesis is easier to be done rather than to accept the alternative (logic of falsification). Rejecting the null hypothesis will bring us closer to accept the alternative hypothesis. For example, it is difficult to prove that **all swans are white**. How many white swans we need to collect to prove that they are all white? But by stating that **not all swans are white**, we only need to show one black swan (or any colour, other than white) to reject that statement.

2.2.4 Set a Criterion to Decide

The criterion normally used in statistics is the level of significance for the test. The significance value normally used is P value or the probability to make Type 1 error, i.e. rejecting H_o when it is true (Fig. 2.5).

So we want smallest P value possible. This is also known as alpha value. When we decide to reject or not to reject H_o, the P value is usually set below 0.05 (or 5 %).[1] This value means that the probability to make Type 1 error is less than 5 %. If the probability to make error is less than 5 % than we will reject H_o. We have less error, so we have more evidence to reject the H_o. If $P > 0.05$, we cannot reject the H_o.

We use reject or **not reject**, instead of reject and accept the Ho. This is very philosophical. In court when someone is charged with any misconduct, the 'hypothesis' is, "he is not guilty (until proven otherwise)". If the evidence is sufficient (beyond reasonable doubt), the judge (or jury in some countries) will issue a guilty verdict which is actually rejecting the hypothesis of not guilty. However, if

[1]This value is suggested by Fisher (Fisher 1925) as a convenient cut-off point to judge whether a deviation is significant or not. It is just a suggestion but been taken as standard criterion by the mass.

the evidence is insufficient, the hypothesis stays. The persecutor's job is to prove that he is guilty, if they failed, then the presumption of not guilty prevails. The judge can declare not guilty but not innocence.

2.2.5 *Choosing Suitable Statistical Test*

Next is to choose suitable statistical test to test the hypothesis. The choice of test depends on:

1. Objective of the test
2. Level of measurements for dependent and independent variable
3. Number of dependent and independent variable
4. Distribution of the numerical measures whether Normal or not

Table 2.2 How to choose statistical test

Dependant (outcome) variable	Independent variable	Test
One sample		
Numerical normal	N/A	One-sample t-test
Numerical not normal	N/A	Wilcoxon signed-rank test
Categorical	N/A	χ^2-goodness of fit
Unpaired variables		
Categorical	Categorical	χ^2 test or Fisher's exact test
Categorical 2 categories	Numerical normal	Independent sample t-test
Categorical 2 categories	Numerical not normal	Mann–Whitney U or log rank test
Categorical > 2 categories	Numerical normal	Logistic regression*
Categorical > 2 categories	Numerical not normal	Logistic regression*
Numerical normal	Categorical > 2 categories	One-way ANOVA
Numerical normal	Numerical normal	Pearson Correlation Coefficient test
Numerical normal	Numerical not normal	Spearman Correlation Coefficient test
Numerical not normal	Categorical	Kruskall–Wallis test
Numerical not normal	Numerical normal	Spearman Correlation Coefficient test
Numerical not normal	Numerical not normal	Spearman Correlation Coefficient test
Paired variables		
Categorical	Categorical	McNemar test
Numerical normal	Numerical normal	Paired t-test
Numerical not normal	Numerical not normal	Wilcoxon signed-rank test

*If you wish just to test for significance difference, maybe you could categorise the variable and use χ^2 test instead

There are already many tables, guidelines, graphics and algorithms on how to choose correct statistical test. This book provides just a simple guideline in Table 2.2. Readers are encourage to read further.

2.2.6 *Making a Decision*

The test will provide us with P value. We then need to compare the P value with the cut-off point that we chose before we analyse the data. If we use P value < 0.05 as the cut-off point, when the test $P < 0.05$ we will reject the H_o and the conclusion should be that whatever difference we observed is significant.

In the subsequent chapters, step-by-step description on most of the bivariable analyses will be showed; and from Sect. 2.6 onwards, description and guide on multivariable analyses will follow.

2.3 Comparing Means

2.3.1 *Compare One Mean*

Using Data 2.1 above, if we wish to compare the mean BMI that was observed with values previously measured (24.37 kg/m^2) (Azmi et al. 2009) we could use **one-sample t-test.**

SPSS Analysis: One-Sample T-test

1. Click Analyse
2. Click Compare Means
3. Click One-Sample T Test
4. Move 'bmi' to Test variable(s) box
5. Enter 24.37 (which was obtained from other study) into Test Value box
6. Click OK

SPSS Output

The analysis showed that BMI observed in this study (25.81 kg/m^2) is significantly higher ($P < 0.001$)[2] compared to the mean BMI from Azmi MY et al. 2009 (24.37 kg/m^2) (Azmi et al. 2009)

[2]Never write $P = 0.000$ because it is meaningless. It has a value but too small for SPSS to display it. The correct way to describe it is by stating the P-value as $P < 0.001$.

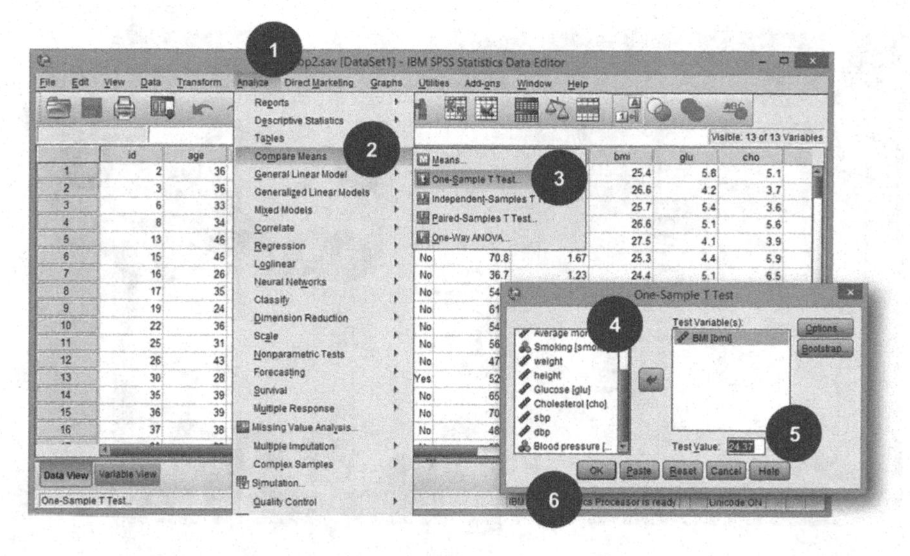

Screen 2.4 Testing one mean to a known value using One-sample t-test

One-Sample Statistics

	N	Mean	Std. Deviation	Std. Error Mean
BMI	150	25.812	2.2614	.1846

One-Sample Test

	Test Value = 24.37					
					95% Confidence Interval of the Difference	
	t	df	Sig. (2-tailed)	Mean Difference	Lower	Upper
BMI	7.811	149	.000	1.4422	1.077	1.807

Output 2.7 Comparing one mean to a known value

2.3.2 Compare Two Means

Using Data 2.1, if we like to compare means of plasma glucose (in mmol/L) between male and female, we could use Independent sample t-test.

SPSS Analysis: Independent sample T-test

1. Click Analyse
2. Click Compare Means
3. Click Independent Samples T-Test
4. Move Glucose to Test Variable(s) box
5. Move gender to Grouping Variable box

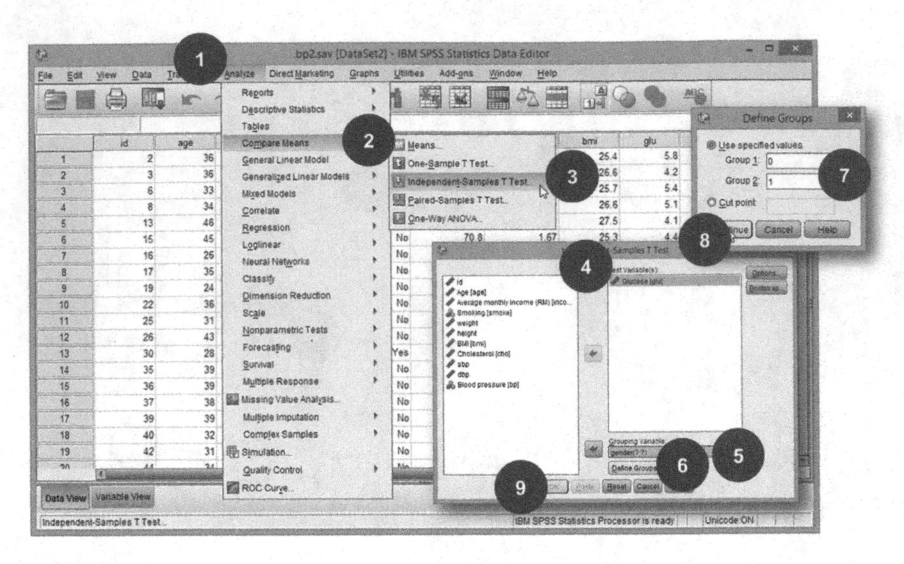

Screen 2.5 How to compare two means using Independent sample t-test

6. Click Define Groups
7. Type 0 for Group 1 and 1 for Group 2 (because the code for gender is 0 = Female, 1 = Male)
8. Click Continue
9. Finally, click OK

SPSS Output

The first table (Group Statistics) describes the summary of means between male and female. It shows that the mean of glucose for female is just slightly higher than for male (5.6 vs. 5.5 mmol). Since Levene's Test for Equality of Variances shows P = 0.065,[3] we can assume that variances are equal. Therefore, observe the

Group Statistics

	Gender	N	Mean	Std. Deviation	Std. Error Mean
Glucose	Female	83	5.633	1.3826	.1518
	Male	67	5.488	1.2644	.1545

Independent Samples Test

		Levene's Test for Equality of Variances		t-test for Equality of Means					95% Confidence Interval of the Difference	
		F	Sig.	t	df	Sig. (2-tailed)	Mean Difference	Std. Error Difference	Lower	Upper
Glucose	Equal variances assumed	3.459	.065	.664	148	.508	.1451	.2186	-.2869	.5772
	Equal variances not assumed			.670	145.665	.504	.1451	.2165	-.2829	.5731

Output 2.8 Comparing two means

[3]The H_o for Levene's Test is that there is no difference of variances between the groups. If P > 0.05, we could not reject the H_o, and therefore the variances can be assumed as equal.

statistical values in the first row where the P value for the t-test is 0.508. This means that there is no significant difference in means of blood glucose between male and female.

2.3.3 Compare More Than Two Means

When we have more than two means to compare, we should use Analysis of Variance (ANOVA). We should not do multiple t-tests because that will increase the possibility of making Type-1 error. In Data 2.1, we can compare means of blood glucose (in mmol/L) between three different BMI statuses. If we use recommended BMI action level for Asian (WHO 2003), we could classify BMI into three categories: Normal (below 23 kg/m^2), Overweight (23 until below 27.5 kg/m^2) and Obese (27.5 kg/m^2 and above). We use Visual binning in SPSS to transform a numerical data into categorical.

SPSS Transform: Visual Binning

1. Click Transform
2. Click Visual Binning
3. Move BMI to Variables to Bin
4. Click Continue
5. Type a name for the new variable (e.g. bmistat)
6. Type a label (e.g. BMI Status)
7. For Row 1, enter 23 in the Value, then Normal as the Label; 27.5 and Overweight for Row 2 and leave HIGH in Row 3, type Obese for the Label.
8. Check Exclude in the Upper Endpoints
9. Click OK
10. Confirm to create a new variable by clicking OK when prompted.

We will get a new variable (Screen 2.7) located at the end of the list. We will now able to compare the means of glucose.

SPSS Analysis: One-way ANOVA

1. Click Analyze
2. Click Compare Means
3. Click One-Way ANOVA
4. Move Glucose to Dependence List
5. Move BMI Status to Factor
6. Click Options. Check Descriptive and Homogeneity of variance test. Then click Continue.

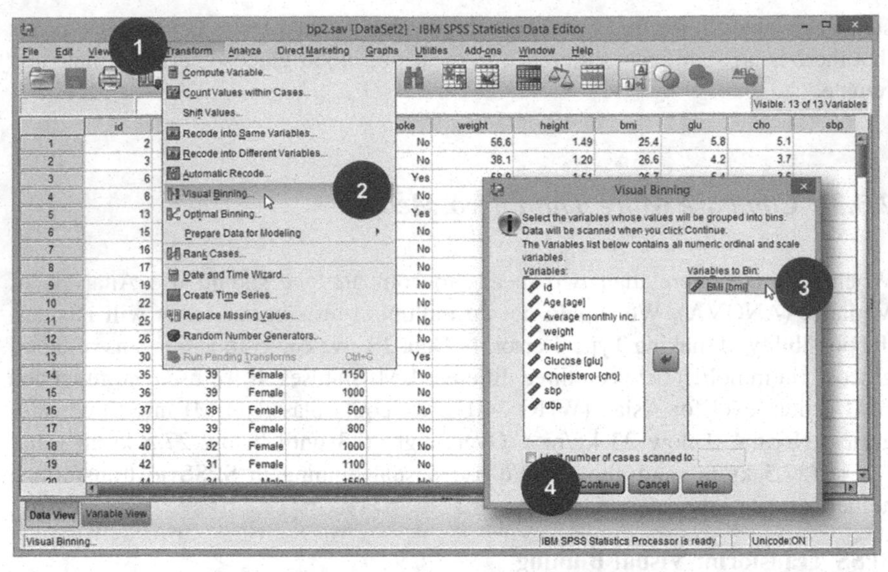

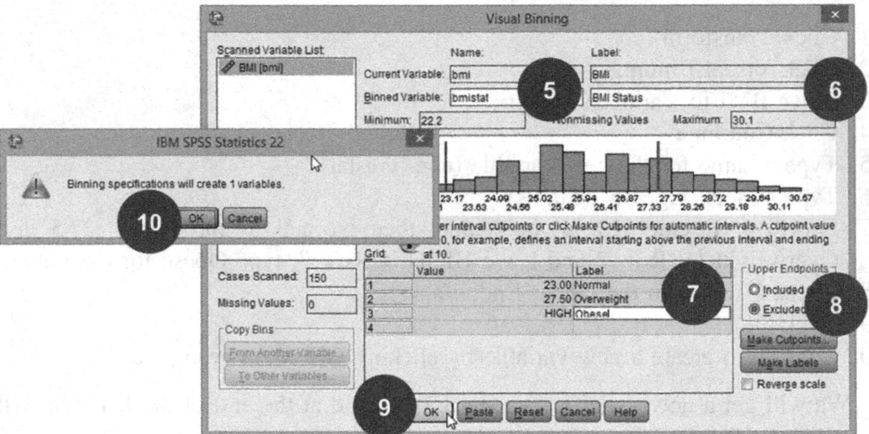

Screen 2.6 Categorising numerical variable using Visual Binning

7. Click Post Hoc. Based on the result of Homogeneity of variance test later, choose appropriate Post Hoc test.[4] Click Continue.
8. Click OK

SPSS Output

The means of glucose for Normal and Overweight were about the same: 5.3 (1.4) mmol/L and 5.4 (1.3) mmol/L, respectively; and Obese subjects have mean of 6.3 (1.3) mmol/L. The difference was significant (F(df = 2, 147) = 6.960, P = 0.01). This indicates that there would be **at least one significant** difference from three possible comparisons (Normal–Overweight, Normal–Obese and Overweight–Obese). Since Levene's statistics indicated that the equal variances can be assumed (P > 0.05), therefore, we could use any of the post hoc test listed under Equal Variances Assumed to determine which comparison is different significantly. In the example above, we used Scheffe's test. The test revealed that the actual different was between Normal–Obese and Overweight–Obese (P = 0.030 and P = 0.002, respectively).

*bp2.sav [DataSet2] - IBM SPSS Statistics Data Editor

File Edit View Data Transform Analyze Direct Marketing Graphs Utilities Add-ons Window Help

Visible: 14 of 14 Variables

	moke	weight	height	bmi	glu	chu	sbp	dbp	bp	bmistat	var
1	No	56.6	1.49	25.4	5.8	5.1	121	74	Normal	Overweight	
2	No	38.1	1.20	26.6	4.2	3.7	117	71	Normal	Overweight	
3	Yes	58.9	1.51	25.7	5.4	3.6	114	77	Normal	Overweight	
4	No	59.1	1.49	26.6	5.1	5.6	117	80	Normal	Overweight	
5	Yes	64.7	1.53	27.5	4.1	3.9	117	75	Normal	Obese	
6	No	70.8	1.67	25.3	4.4	5.9	141	96	High	Overweight	
7	No	36.7	1.23	24.4	5.1	6.5	133	79	Normal	Overweight	
8	No	54.2	1.50	24.2	4.6	3.4	89	62	Normal	Overweight	
9	No	61.9	1.53	26.6	4.5	4.4	113	84	Normal	Overweight	
10	No	54.6	1.47	25.3	4.5	5.3	112	63	Normal	Overweight	
11	No	56.9	1.52	24.5	5.0	5.0	103	81	Normal	Overweight	
12	No	47.7	1.36	25.9	4.1	4.7	107	80	Normal	Overweight	
13	Yes	52.9	1.41	26.4	5.3	5.1	122	73	Normal	Overweight	
14	No	65.8	1.60	25.7	4.4	5.0	121	95	High	Overweight	
15	No	70.5	1.70	24.5	4.2	4.4	115	77	Normal	Overweight	
16	No	48.0	1.34	26.8	4.5	3.2	99	81	Normal	Overweight	
17	No	53.3	1.55	22.2	4.0	6.2	105	79	Normal	Normal	
18	No	51.2	1.43	24.9	4.5	6.9	135	91	High	Overweight	
19	No	37.5	1.25	24.1	4.4	2.1	114	66	Normal	Overweight	

Data View Variable View

IBM SPSS Statistics Processor is ready Unicode:ON

Screen 2.7 A new variable is created after Visual Binning done

[4]When comparing more than two means, ANOVA will turn significant when there is at least two means that differ significantly but since it is an omnibus test, it would not be able to tell which of the means are different. Post hoc test would be able to help us on this. However, there is no one best post hoc test. So any test is acceptable.

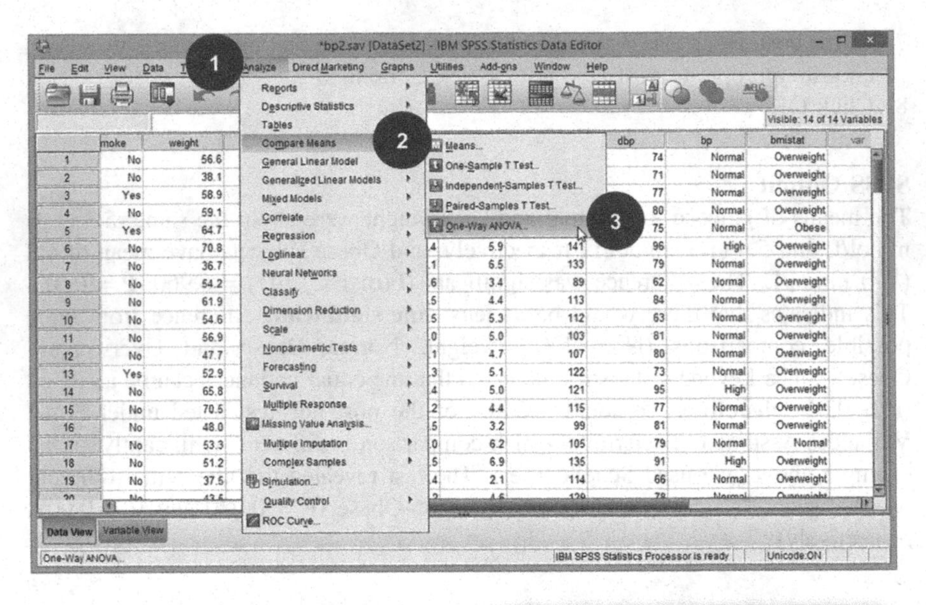

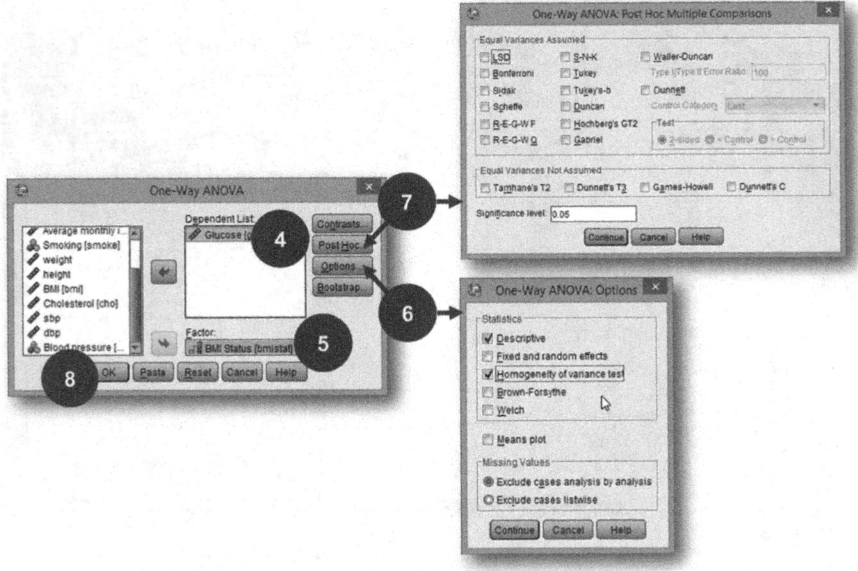

Screen 2.8 Compare means using One-way ANOVA

Descriptives

Glucose

	N	Mean	Std. Deviation	Std. Error	95% Confidence Interval for Mean		Minimum	Maximum
					Lower Bound	Upper Bound		
Normal	17	5.265	1.3540	.3284	4.569	5.961	4.0	8.2
Overweight	99	5.374	1.2634	.1270	5.122	5.626	4.0	11.8
Obese	34	6.285	1.2854	.2204	5.836	6.733	4.1	9.3
Total	150	5.568	1.3287	.1085	5.354	5.783	4.0	11.8

Test of Homogeneity of Variances

Glucose

Levene Statistic	df1	df2	Sig.
.722	2	147	.487

ANOVA

Glucose

	Sum of Squares	df	Mean Square	F	Sig.
Between Groups	22.753	2	11.377	6.960	.001
Within Groups	240.286	147	1.635		
Total	263.039	149			

Output 2.9 Descriptive statistics and ANOVA analysis

Multiple Comparisons

Dependent Variable: Glucose

Scheffe

(I) BMI Status	(J) BMI Status	Mean Difference (I-J)	Std. Error	Sig.	95% Confidence Interval	
					Lower Bound	Upper Bound
Normal	Overweight	-.1094	.3357	.948	-.939	.721
	Obese	-1.0201*	.3798	.030	-1.959	-.081
Overweight	Normal	.1094	.3357	.948	-.721	.939
	Obese	-.9106*	.2541	.002	-1.539	-.282
Obese	Normal	1.0201*	.3798	.030	.081	1.959
	Overweight	.9106*	.2541	.002	.282	1.539

*. The mean difference is significant at the 0.05 level.

Glucose

Scheffe[a,b]

BMI Status	N	Subset for alpha = 0.05	
		1	2
Normal	17	5.265	
Overweight	99	5.374	
Obese	34		6.285
Sig.		.946	1.000

Means for groups in homogeneous subsets are displayed.

a. Uses Harmonic Mean Sample Size = 30.508.

b. The group sizes are unequal. The harmonic mean of the group sizes is used. Type I error levels are not guaranteed.

Output 2.10 Post hoc test result

This data consist of 150 subjects whom blood pressure were tested before and after 6 months weight management programme. Their weight (in kg) and blood pressure status before and after the intervention were recorded.

Data 2.2 Weight management programme

2.3.4 Compare Paired Means

Independent sample t-test and one-way ANOVA are tests to be used when we compare independent[5] means. When the means are dependent, or paired, those tests are no longer appropriate. In Data 2.2, 150 subjects underwent a 6-month weight reduction programme. Their body weight after the programme is very much affected by the weight before the start of intervention.

To compare the weight before and after the programme, we should use paired t-test.[6]

SPSS Analysis: Paired T-test

1. Click Analyze
2. Click Compare Means
3. Click Paired-Samples T Test
4. Move Body weight before to Variable 1 Pair 1 and Body weight after to Variable 2 Pair 1
5. Click OK

SPSS Output

The mean body weight reduced from 53.8 to 51.6 kg. The difference of 2.2 (0.5) kg was significant ($P < 0.001$)

[5]Independent relationship here means that the measurement of one variable is not predetermined by another one, for example, body weight and sex. However, if we are comparing body weight of the same group of people before and after certain health and lifestyle intervention, their body weight after intervention should be affected by their prior weight. Their post-intervention weight is dependent on the weight before the intervention.

[6]Here, we are comparing two dependent measurements. If we wish to measure more than two measurements, we should use Repeated Measure ANOVA (Sect. 2.7).

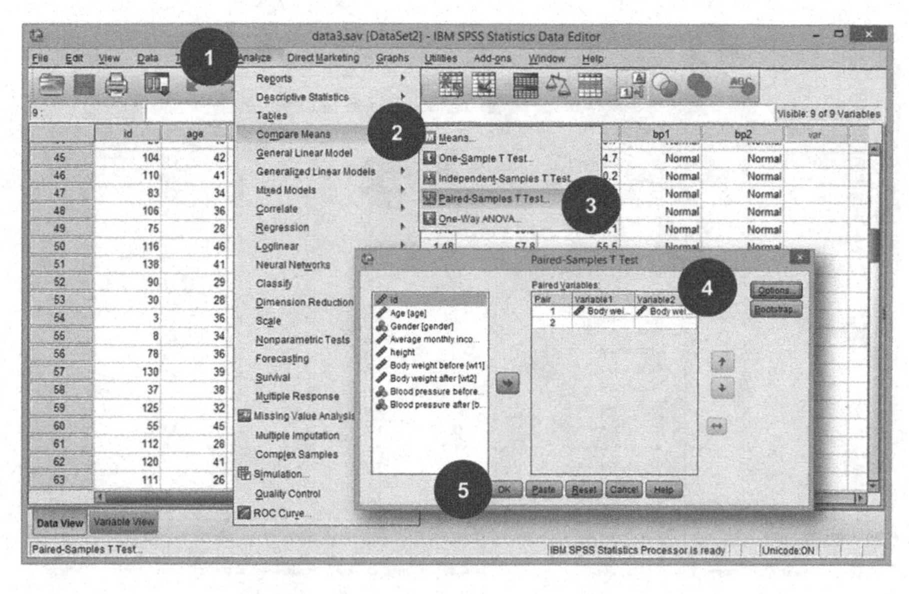

Screen 2.9 Comparing paired means using paired t-test

Paired Samples Statistics

		Mean	N	Std. Deviation	Std. Error Mean
Pair 1	Body weight before	53.814	150	9.4611	.7717
	Body weight after	51.606	150	9.4158	.7688

Paired Samples Correlations

		N	Correlation	Sig.
Pair 1	Body weight before & Body weight after	150	.999	.000

Paired Samples Test

		Paired Differences					t	df	Sig. (2-tailed)
		Mean	Std. Deviation	Std. Error Mean	95% Confidence Interval of the Difference Lower	Upper			
Pair 1	Body weight before - Body weight after	2.2076	.4988	.0407	2.1272	2.2881	54.210	149	.000

Output 2.11 Result from paired t-test

2.4 Comparing Proportions

2.4.1 Compare Independent Proportions

If we wish to test difference of proportions, we could use chi-square test.[7] Using the Data 2.1, we could test differences of proportion of high blood pressure between different BMI status.

[7]The symbol for chi-square is χ^2; not X^2.

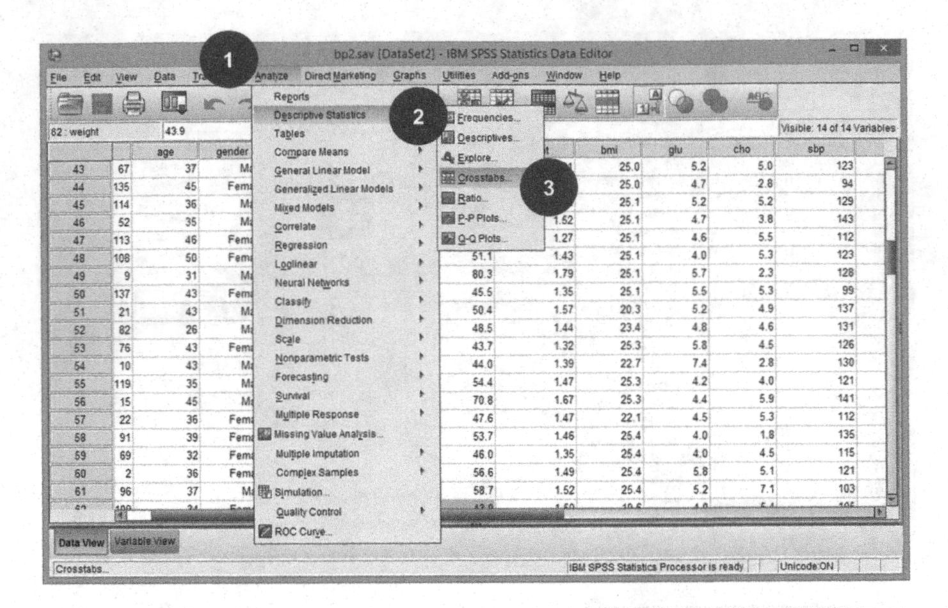

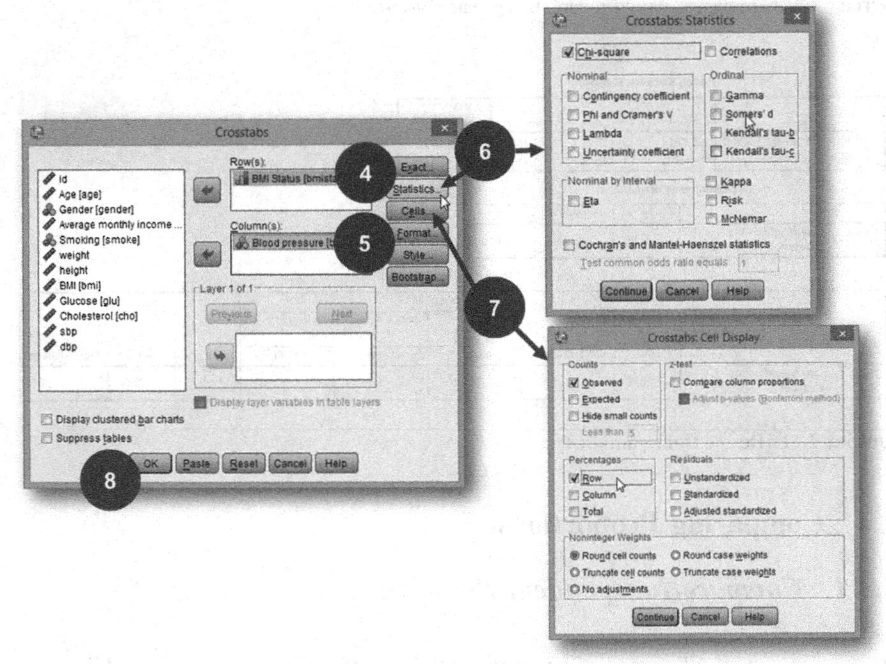

Screen 2.10 Comparing proportions using chi-square test

Case Processing Summary

	Cases					
	Valid		Missing		Total	
	N	Percent	N	Percent	N	Percent
BMI Status * Blood pressure	150	100.0%	0	0.0%	150	100.0%

BMI Status * Blood pressure Crosstabulation

			Blood pressure		Total
			Normal	High	
BMI Status	Normal	Count	10	7	17
		% within BMI Status	58.8%	41.2%	100.0%
	Overweight	Count	54	45	99
		% within BMI Status	54.5%	45.5%	100.0%
	Obese	Count	8	26	34
		% within BMI Status	23.5%	76.5%	100.0%
Total		Count	72	78	150
		% within BMI Status	48.0%	52.0%	100.0%

Chi-Square Tests

	Value	df	Asymp. Sig. (2-sided)
Pearson Chi-Square	10.654[a]	2	.005
Likelihood Ratio	11.145	2	.004
Linear-by-Linear Association	8.371	1	.004
N of Valid Cases	150		

a. 0 cells (0.0%) have expected count less than 5. The minimum expected count is 8.16.

Output 2.12 Result of chi-square test

SPSS Analysis: Chi-square test

1. Click Analyze
2. Click Descriptive Statistics
3. Click Crosstabs
4. Move BMI Status to Rows(s)
5. Move Blood pressure to Column(s)[8]
6. Click Statistics. Check Chi-square. Then click Continue
7. Click Cells. Check Row. Then click Continue
8. Click OK

[8]It does not really matter which variable to put in Row or Column, but it would be recommended to put dependant variable in the Column. Then it would make sense to Request Row Percent in Step 7. We will then compare High Blood Pressure between Normal, Overweight and Obese category.

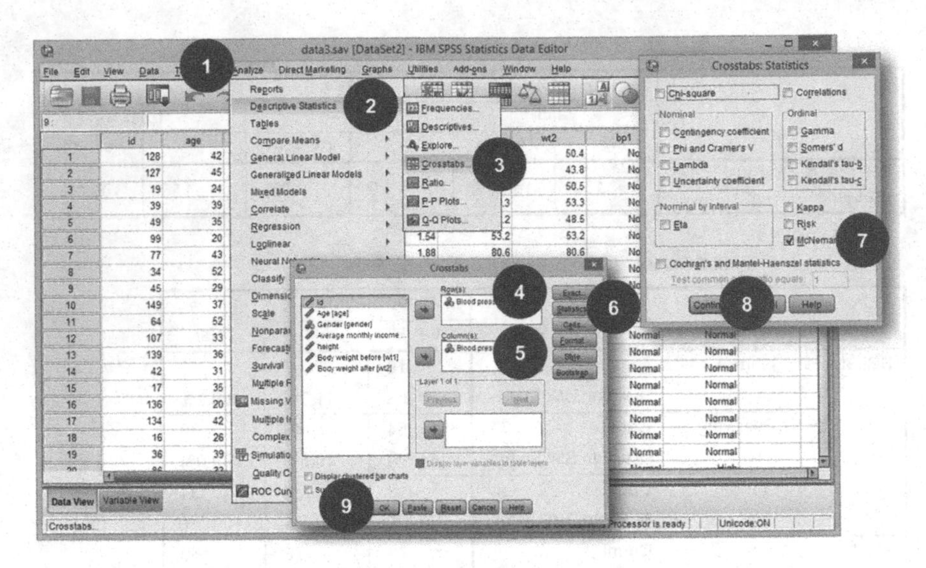

Screen 2.11 Comparing paired proportions using McNemar test

Case Processing Summary

	Cases					
	Valid		Missing		Total	
	N	Percent	N	Percent	N	Percent
Blood pressure before * Blood pressure after	150	100.0%	0	0.0%	150	100.0%

Blood pressure before * Blood pressure after Crosstabulation

			Blood pressure after		Total
			Normal	High	
Blood pressure before	Normal	Count	69	3	72
		% within Blood pressure before	95.8%	4.2%	100.0%
	High	Count	29	49	78
		% within Blood pressure before	37.2%	62.8%	100.0%
Total		Count	98	52	150
		% within Blood pressure before	65.3%	34.7%	100.0%

Chi-Square Tests

	Value	Exact Sig. (2-sided)
McNemar Test		.000[a]
N of Valid Cases	150	

a. Binomial distribution used.

Output 2.13 Result for McNemar test

SPSS Output
It was pretty obvious that the proportion of Obese group who had high blood pressure was higher (76.5 %) compared to both Normal and Overweight groups. The difference was significant (χ^2 (df = 2) = 10.654, P = 0.005).[9]

2.4.2 *Compare Paired Proportions*

Chi-square is chosen when the proportions compared are independent. However, when the proportions are dependent on each other, for instance in Data 2.2, when blood pressures were compared before and after a 6-month weight management programme, we should use McNemar as the proper test.

SPSS Analysis: McNemar Test

1. Click Analyze
2. Click Descriptive Statistics
3. Click Crosstabs
4. Move Blood pressure before into the Rows(s) box
5. Move Blood pressure after into the Column(s) box
6. Click Statistics
7. Check McNemar
8. Click Continue
9. Click OK

SPSS Output
From 78 subjects with high blood pressure initially, 29 (37 %) showed lower blood pressure status after the programme (P < 0.001).

2.5 Comparing Ranks

When testing differences of numerical measures between groups, we could compare the means but if the distribution is not normal, using mean is bias. When we are not able to use mean to describe the data, we also should not compare means for skewed measurements. As mentioned previously, we should use median to describe

[9]Pearson chi-square is not suitable if there are more than 20 % of cells with expected count less than 5. For the above example, it is a 3x2 cells comparison (three groups for BMI status and two groups for hypertension status). If two out of its six cells have small sample size, it is already 33 %. For such instance, exact test is a better alternative.

This is a study on waiting times (in minutes) among 80 patients who attended outpatient clinics divided into Medical and Surgical units in three different settings (primary care, specialist and tertiary).

Data 2.3 Waiting time

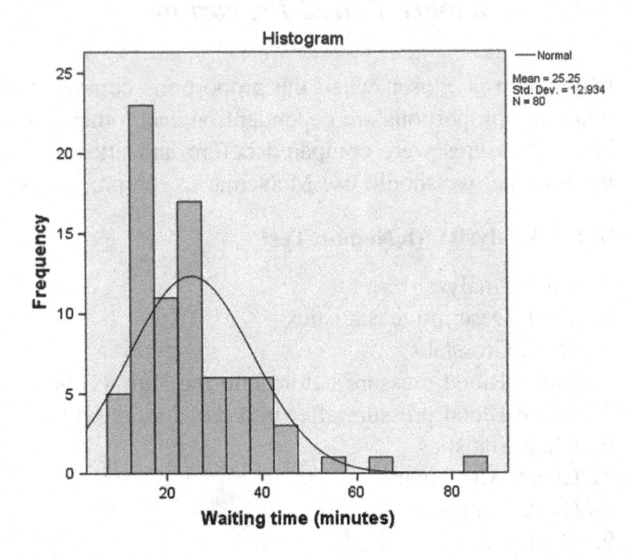

Fig. 2.6 Distribution of waiting time (minutes)

skewed data, but to test whether the difference is significant or not, we should compare the **ranks**[10]. We will be using Data 2.3 to illustrate this method.

When we check the distribution of the waiting time (Fig. 2.6), it is pretty obvious that the data are skewed to the right with mean 25.3 min and median 23 min, ranging from 10 to 84 min.

2.5.1 Compare Two Independent Nonparametric Samples

Mann–Whitney U test is usually used as an alternative to t-test for not normally distributed data. This is suitable when we wish to compare waiting times (which is not normally distributed) between Medical and Surgical clinics.

[10]The data are sorted according to groups from smallest value to the highest. Then the values at the middle of each group are compared. For example, if we compare data such as 10, 20, 20, 30, 40 versus 10, 20, 30, 30, 50, we are actually comparing 20 and 30.

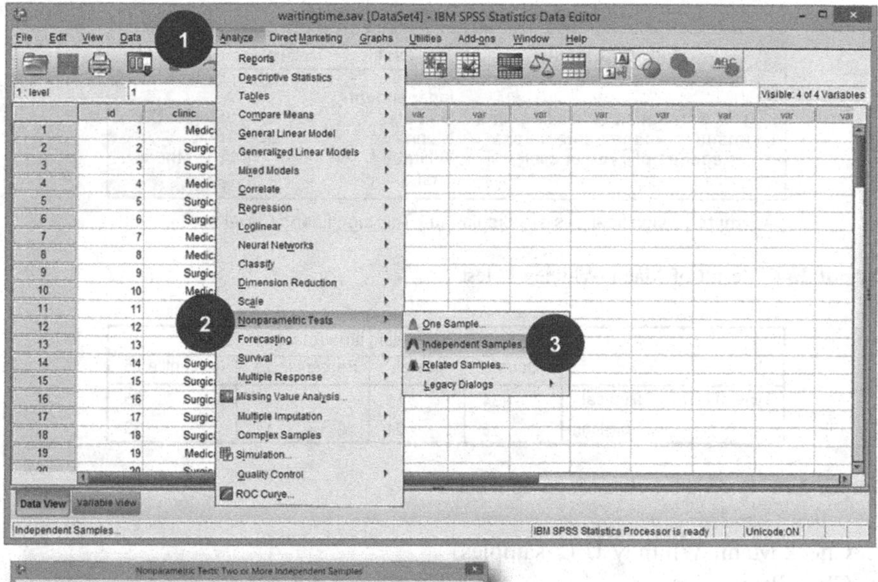

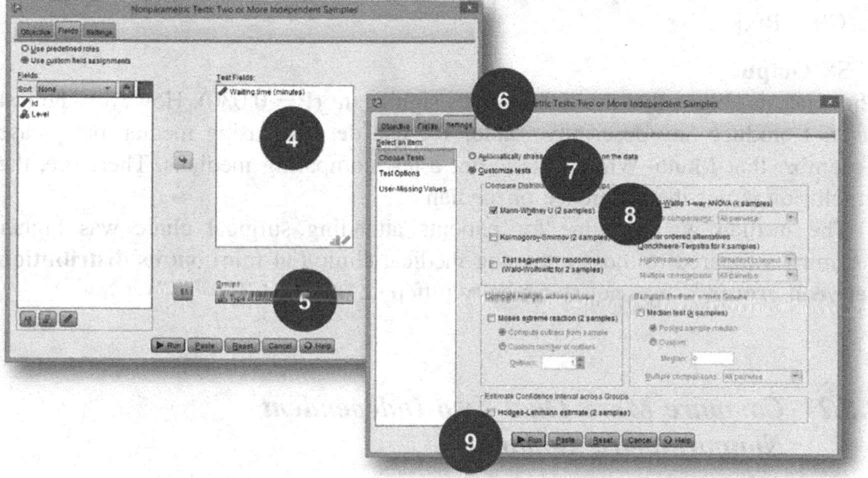

Screen 2.12 Comparing ranks of two independent samples using Mann–Whitney U test

SPSS Analysis: Mann–Whitney U test

1. Click Analyze
2. Click Nonparametric Tests
3. Click Independent Samples
4. Under Fields tab, move Waiting time into Test Fields box
5. Move Type of clinic to Groups box
6. Click Setting tab
7. Check Customize tests

Hypothesis Test Summary

	Null Hypothesis	Test	Sig.	Decision
1	The distribution of Waiting time (minutes) is the same across categories of Type of clinic.	Independent-Samples Mann-Whitney U Test	.030	Reject the null hypothesis.

Asymptotic significances are displayed. The significance level is .05.

Output 2.14 Result of Mann–Whitney U test

		Waiting time (minutes)			
		Count	Median	Percentile 25	Percentile 75
Type of clinic	Medical	34	19	15	25
	Surgical	46	24	17	33

Output 2.15 Descriptive statistics using median

8. Check Mann-Whitney U (2 samples)
9. Click Run

SPSS Output

The analysis shows that the difference is significant (P = 0.030). However, the test did not produce any descriptive table. We can describe using median but please remember that Mann–Whitney U is not a test comparing medians. Therefore, the conclusion is not the difference of median.

The median waiting time for patients attending surgical clinic was higher (46 min) compared to those attending medical clinic (34 min) but its **distribution between groups**[11] was not statistically different.

2.5.2 Compare More Than Two Independent Nonparametric Samples

When we want to compare waiting time between primary care, specialist and tertiary centre, we use Kruskal–Wallis which is the one-way ANOVA equivalent for nonparametric samples.

The steps are similar like for Mann–Whitney U test but instead of choosing Mann–Whitney U we choose Kruskal–Wallis test.

[11]Using distribution between groups rather than median between groups because Mann–Whitney U test does not test difference of medians.

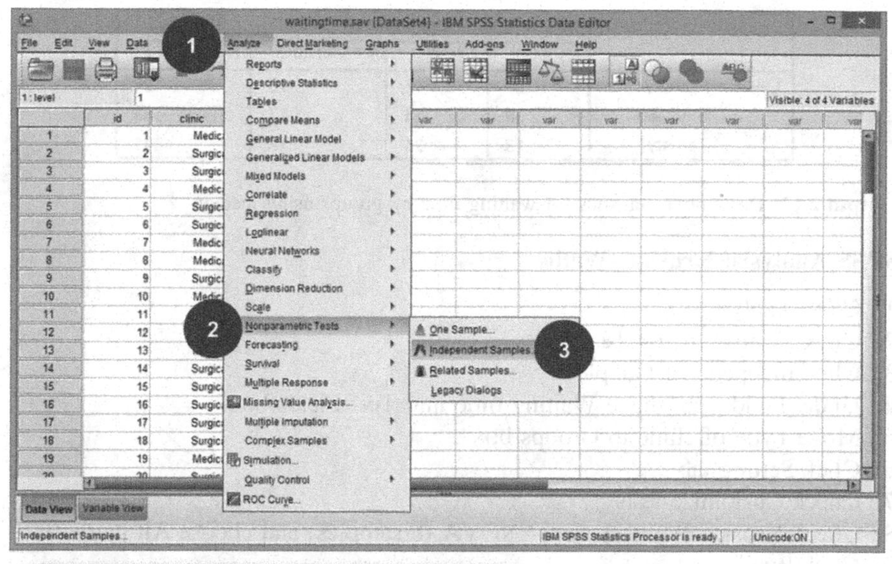

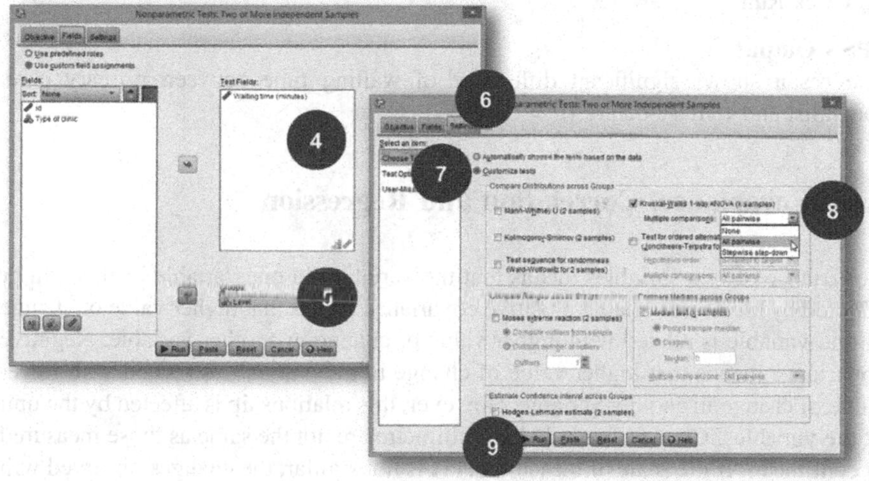

Screen 2.13 Comparing ranks using Kruskal–Wallis test

Hypothesis Test Summary

	Null Hypothesis	Test	Sig.	Decision
1	The distribution of Waiting time (minutes) is the same across categories of Level.	Independent-Samples Kruskal-Wallis Test	.009	Reject the null hypothesis.

Asymptotic significances are displayed. The significance level is .05.

Output 2.16 Result of Kruskal–Wallis test

		Waiting time (minutes)			
		Count	Median	Percentile 25	Percentile 75
Level	Primary care	29	17	13	25
	Specialist	38	24	17	33
	Tertiary	13	24	18	41

Output 2.17 Descriptive statistics for waiting time by groups using median

SPSS Analysis: Kruskal–Wallis

1. Click Analyze
2. Click Nonparametric Tests
3. Click Independent Samples
4. Under Fields tab, move Waiting time into Test Fields box
5. Move Type of clinic to Groups box
6. Click Setting tab
7. Check Customize tests
8. Check Kruskal-Wallis 1-way ANOVA (k samples) and choose All pairwise
9. Click Run

SPSS Output
The result shows significant difference of waiting time between primary care, specialist and tertiary centre (P = 0.009).

2.6 Covariance, Correlation and Regression

Covariance of two variables means that the variation in one variable is affecting or affected by the other variable. Positive covariance means that higher value of change in one variable is related with higher value of change in another variable. Negative covariance means that higher value of change in one variable is related with lower value of change in another variable. However, this relationship is affected by the unit of the variables. Changes recorded in millimetre are not the same as those measured in centimetre. If the scale of measurements is not similar, the changes observed will be different. To measure the change properly, it has to be standardised.

Correlation is the standardised covariance ranging with value from −1 to 1. Correlation measures linear relationship between two numerical variables, i.e. how changes in one variable affect the changes in the other variable (Fig. 2.7).

2.6.1 Correlation Coefficient Test

Using Data 2.4, we would like to test correlation between HbA1c (in %) and systolic blood pressure (mmHg). Theoretically, lower HbA1c indicates good diabetic control. So we would expect positive correlation between HbA1c and SBP. The higher the HbA1c (means poor control), the higher the blood pressure.

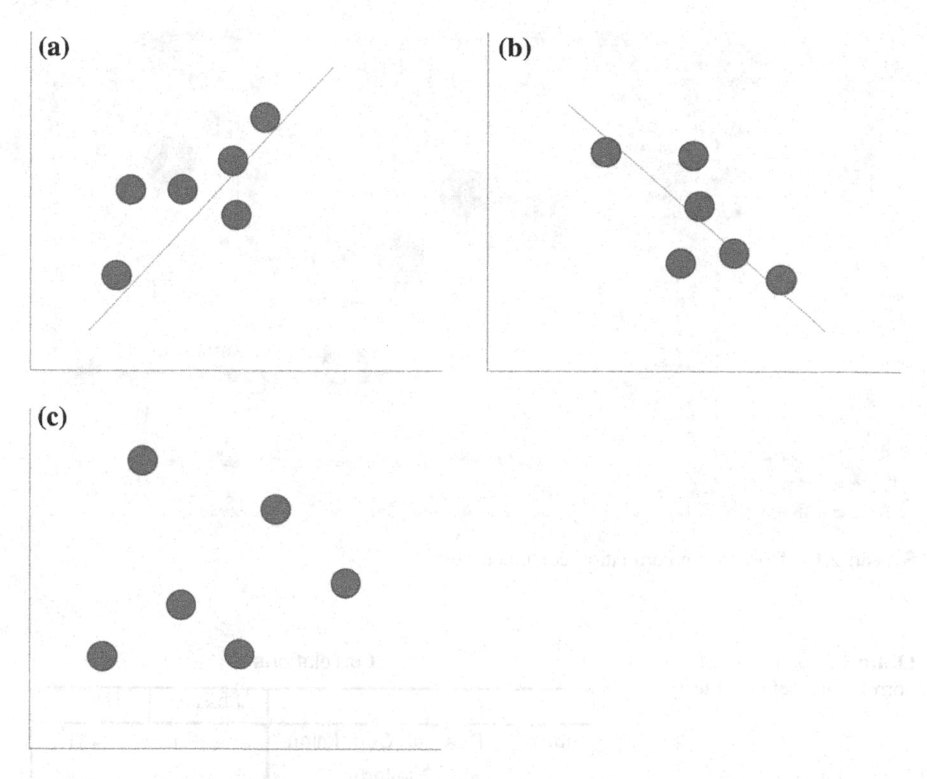

Fig. 2.7 Correlation. **a** Strong positive correlation, **b** strong negative correlation, **c** no linear correlation

A study on diabetic control (HbA1c in %) of sixty patients and its relationship with systolic blood pressure (SBP) (mmHg).

Data 2.4 Diabetic control and hypertension

SPSS Analysis: Correlation coefficient test

1. Click Analyze
2. Click Correlate
3. Click Bivariate
4. Move both hba1c and sbp into Variables box
5. Pearson (correlation test) already checked by default. You can check Spearman if one or both of the variables are not Normal
6. Click OK

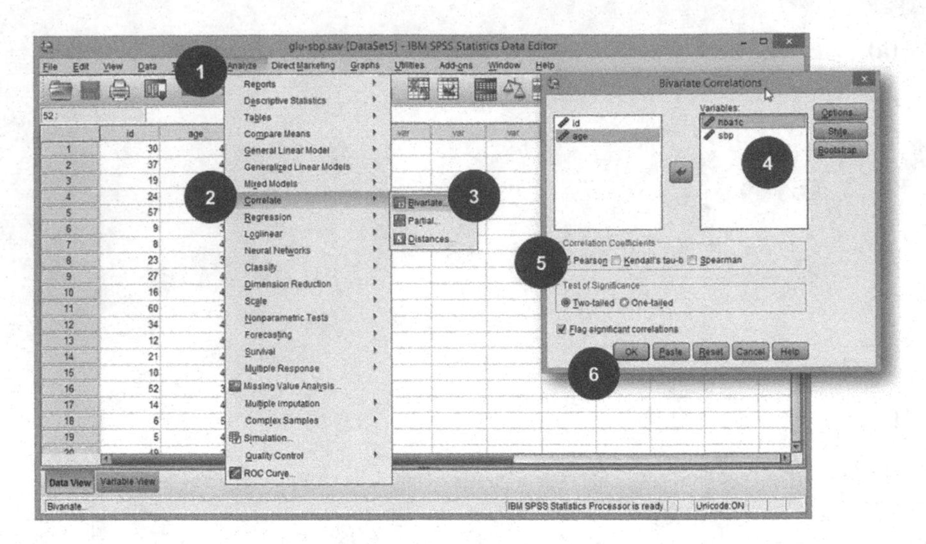

Screen 2.14 How to run correlation coefficient test

Output 2.18 Result of correlation coefficient test

Correlations

		hba1c	sbp
hba1c	Pearson Correlation	1	.431**
	Sig. (2-tailed)		.001
	N	60	60
sbp	Pearson Correlation	.431**	1
	Sig. (2-tailed)	.001	
	N	60	60

**. Correlation is significant at the 0.01 level (2-tailed).

SPSS Output

There is a significant moderate[12] positive correlation between HbA1c and SBP ($r = 0.431$, $P = 0.001$).

2.6.2 *Simple and Multiple Linear Regression*

Regression means the process of fitting all observed data into a line. It takes the relationship of two variables to the next level. Instead of just looking at changes

[12]Usually, the cut-off point for interpretation is as follows: Weak 0.1–0.3, Moderate 0.4–0.7 and Strong ≥ 0.8 regardless of direction (positive or negative).

Fig. 2.8 Linear regression

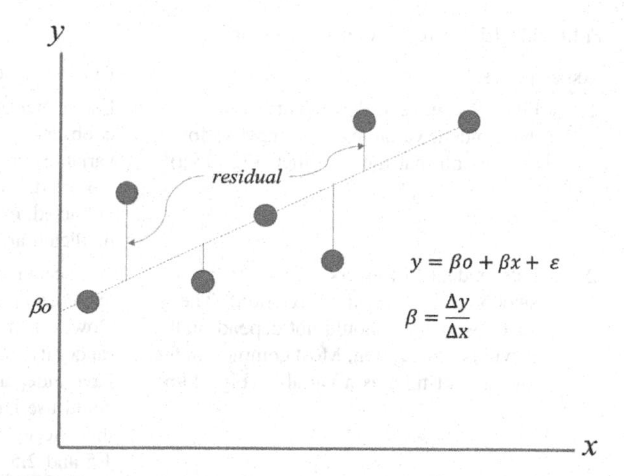

between two variables, it will also describe the direction of change. If we are looking at the relationship between variable A and B, A causing B is not the same as B causing A. One would be the dependent variable and the other one as independent variable. If A is causing B, then A is the independent variable and B is the dependent variable. B depends on A to happen.

In linear regression, a straight line is drawn to represent all the observations (Fig. 2.8). It is summarised as equation $y = \beta_0 + \beta x + \varepsilon$, where y is the dependent variable, x is the independent variable and ε is the residuals (errors) of the regression. β_o is the constant or the intercept, i.e. y value when $x = 0$; and β is the coefficient of x. Pay particular attention to the residuals (errors). **Residuals are the difference between predicted y (using the equation) and observed y at given x.** If the model is good, the total difference should be low, meaning that the model predicts observed values very well.

If there is only one independent variable, we call the model as simple linear regression. When we have two or more independent variables, we call it multiple linear regression. For multiple linear regression with two independents, the equation is $y = \beta o + \beta_1 x_1 + \beta_2 x_2 + \varepsilon$, where x_1 and x_2 are the two different variables.

There are few important assumptions to be adhered to when using linear regression which include linearity between dependant variable and the predictors (independent variables), independence of observations, homogeneity of variance, absence of multicollinearity and normality of errors (Table 2.3).

> A study to determine the relationship of physical activity measured in total weekly energy expenditure from leisure-time physical activities for each individual in metabolic equivalents-hours (MET-Hr) for 58 diabetic patients. Diabetic control was measured using HbA1c (%). Confounders include age, sex and BMI (kg/m^2).

Data 2.5 Diabetic control and physical activity

Table 2.3 Linear regression assumptions

Assumptions		Diagnostics check
1.	Linearity between dependent and independent variables—the most serious assumption that must be met (Fig. 2.9a)	Use scatter plot to check that a straight line is observed between dependent and variables or no obvious patterned observed when plotting observed versus predicted; or diagonal line if residuals and predicted are plotted
2	Independence of errors—no autocorrelation (serial correlation). The next observation should not depend on the previous observation. Most common in the presence of time as a variable (Fig. 2.9b)	Use scatter plot to observe the autocorrelation pattern (Fig. 2.9b). However, if samples are collected randomly, there should be less likely to have independence bias. In SPSS, we could use Durbin–Watson test to verify this. Acceptable range should be within 1.5 and 2.5
3	Homogeneity of variance—the variance should be constant (Fig. 2.9c)	Use scatter plot between standardised residual (y-axis) and standardised predicted (x-axis). The points should be scattered randomly and equally around 0
4	Absence of multicollinearity, i.e. correlation between predictors	Check Tolerance/VIF. If no multicollinearity present, the value should be Tolerance > 0.1 or VIF < 10
5	Normal distribution	Check distribution of the residuals. It should be normal distribution.
6	No outliers or influential point	We can use Casewise Diagnostics and decide the cut-off point for the outliers Cook's distance able to measure the influential points. The maximum value should be < 4/*n*, where n is the sample size Influential observation can also be identified using Leverage Point. Any value bigger than $\frac{2(K+1)}{n}$, where K is the number of predictors and *n* is the sample size, is considered as an influential data

We will use Data 2.5 to analyse the association between diabetic control and physical activity using simple linear regression. It is *simple* because we only consider one predictor in the model (i.e. physical activity). First and foremost, we should check the presence of linearity between HbA1c and MET-Hr. To do that, we will draw a scatter plot.

SPSS Analysis: Scatter Plot

1. Click Graph
2. Click Chart Builder
3. Click Scatter/Dot from the Gallery tab
4. Drag HbA1c to y-axis, MET-Hr to x-axis
5. Click OK

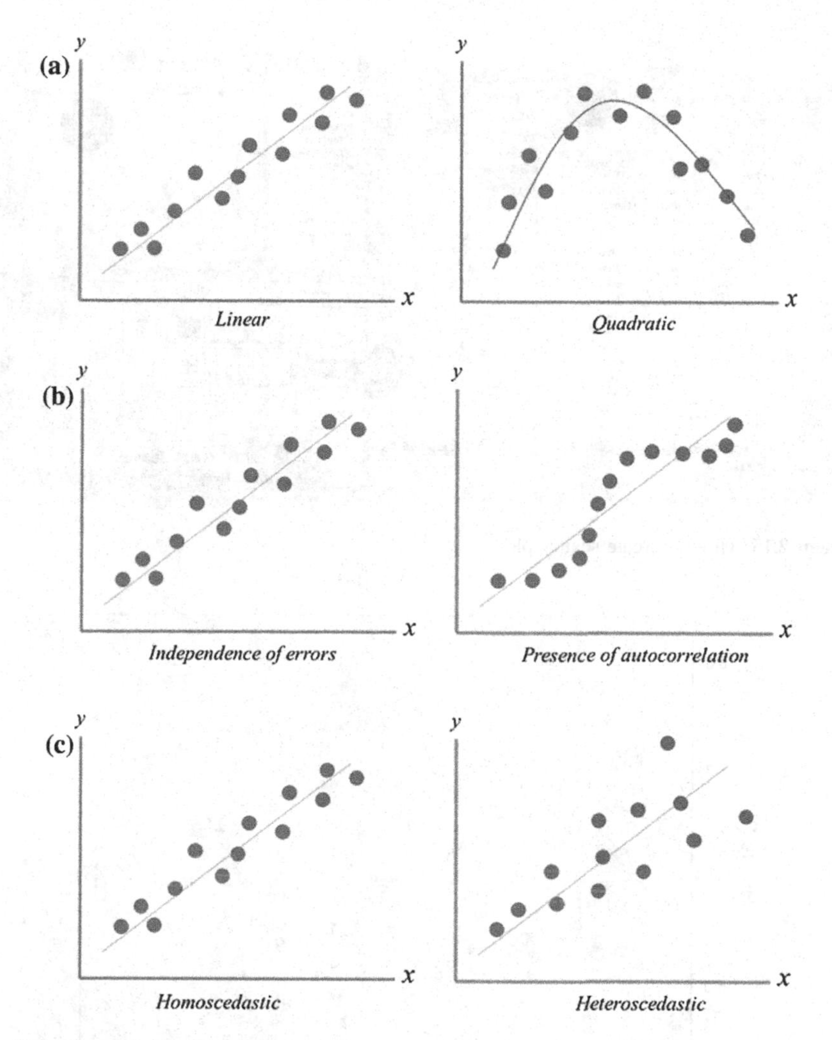

Fig. 2.9 Regression assumptions

SPSS Output

The scatter plot shows evidence of linear association between MET-Hr and HbA1c. Once we have proved that there is indeed a linear association, we can proceed with linear regression.

SPSS Analysis: Simple Linear Regression

1. Click Analyse
2. Click Regression
3. Click Linear
4. Move HbA1c to Dependant box

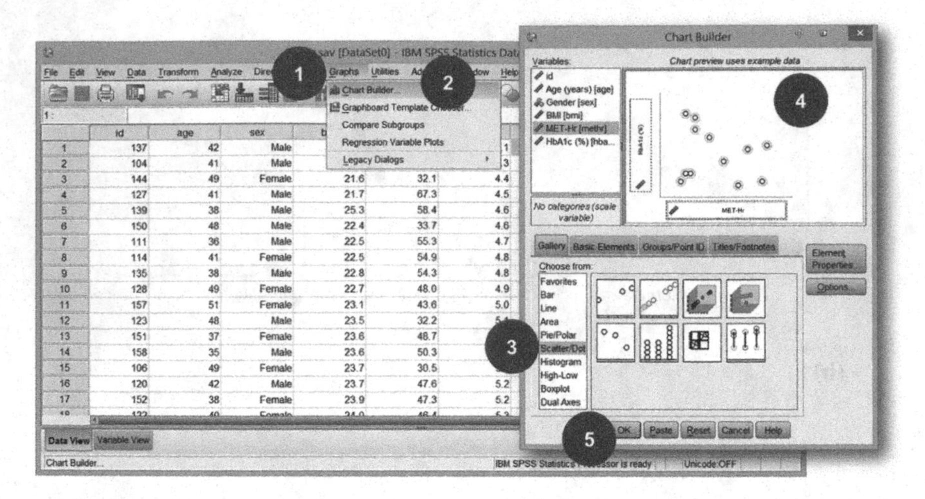

Screen 2.15 How to create scatter plot

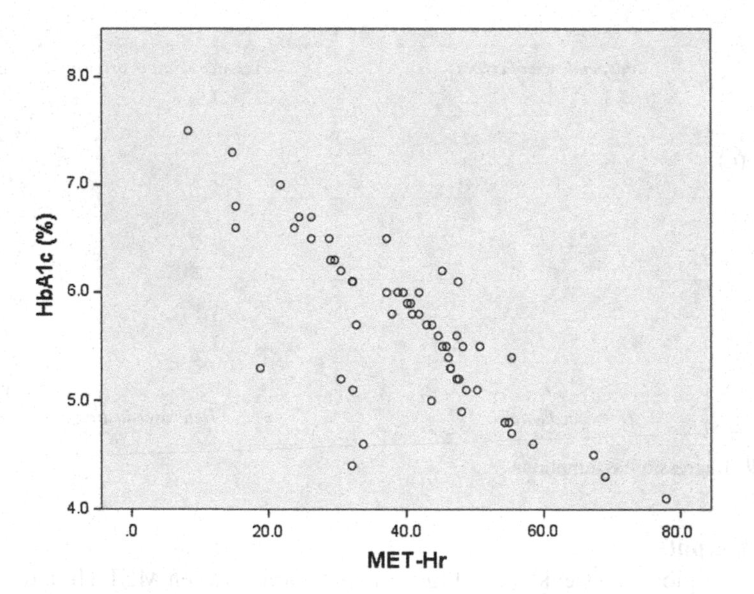

Output 2.19 Scatter plot

5. Move MET-Hr to Independent(s) box
6. Click Statistics
7. Estimates and Model Fit already checked by default. Click Casewise diagnostics to check for outliers. 3 SD was the default. This means anything outside ±3SD will be considered as outlier. You may check Durbin-Watson if you believe there is autocorrelation in your data. You can check Collinearity

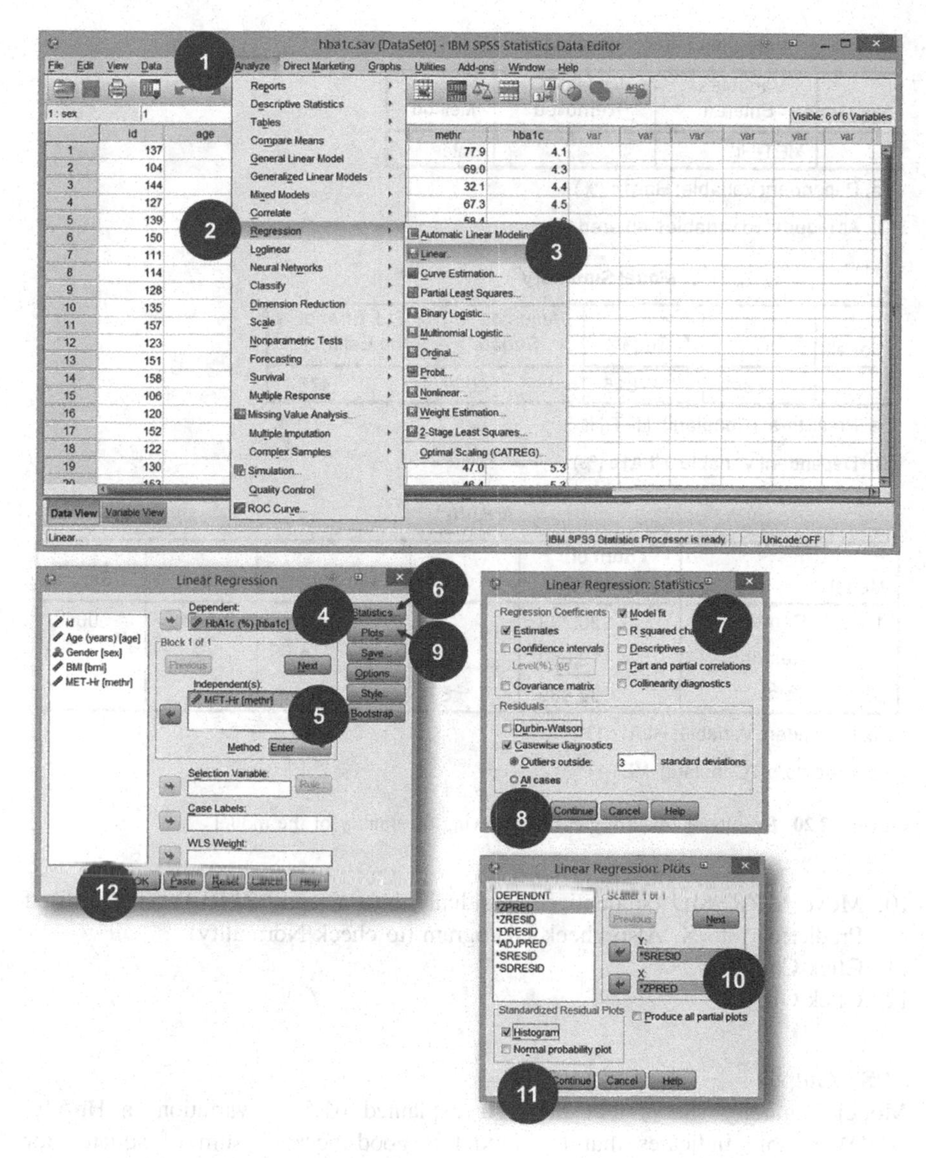

Screen 2.16 How to run Simple Linear Regression

diagnostics if you have more than one predictors in the model, else it is of no use.

8. Click Continue
9. Click Plots

Variables Entered/Removed[a]

Model	Variables Entered	Variables Removed	Method
1	MET-Hr[b]	.	Enter

a. Dependent Variable: HbA1c (%)

b. All requested variables entered.

Model Summary[b]

Model	R	R Square	Adjusted R Square	Std. Error of the Estimate
1	.784[a]	.615	.609	.4753

a. Predictors: (Constant), MET-Hr

b. Dependent Variable: HbA1c (%)

ANOVA[a]

Model		Sum of Squares	df	Mean Square	F	Sig.
1	Regression	20.239	1	20.239	89.601	.000[b]
	Residual	12.650	56	.226		
	Total	32.889	57			

a. Dependent Variable: HbA1c (%)

b. Predictors: (Constant), MET-Hr

Output 2.20 Results of linear regression showing the quality of the model

10. Move *SRRESID (studentized Residuals) into Y and *ZPRED (standardised Predicted) into X. Also check Histogram (to check Normality)
11. Click Continue
12. Click OK

SPSS Output

Model Summary shows that MET-Hr explained 61.5 % variation in HbA1c. ANOVA table indicates that the model is good because sum of squares for regression (20.239) is more than the residuals ($F(1,56) = 89.601$, $P < 0.001$).

Coefficients table is the main table for linear regression. This table shows that HbA1c = 7.425 – 0.044 (MET-Hr), meaning that if we have metabolic hours information, we can predict our HbA1c. MET-Hr is significantly associated with HbA1c. Negative coefficient value indicates that the association is negative. The higher the physical activity, the lower the HbA1c, i.e. better diabetic control.

Casewise Diagnostics suggests that Case Number 3 (row 3 of our dataset) is an outlier. It is good that we investigate this case and decide whether we keep or throw away the data.

Coefficients[a]

Model		Unstandardized Coefficients		Standardized Coefficients	t	Sig.
		B	Std. Error	Beta		
1	(Constant)	7.425	.194		38.271	.000
	MET-Hr	-.044	.005	-.784	-9.466	.000

a. Dependent Variable: HbA1c (%)

Casewise Diagnostics[a]

Case Number	Std. Residual	HbA1c (%)	Predicted Value	Residual
3	-3.417	4.4	6.024	-1.6242

a. Dependent Variable: HbA1c (%)

Output 2.21 Result of linear regression showing the contribution of MET-Hr to the model

Residuals Statistics[a]

	Minimum	Maximum	Mean	Std. Deviation	N
Predicted Value	4.025	7.067	5.686	.5959	58
Std. Predicted Value	-2.787	2.318	.000	1.000	58
Standard Error of Predicted Value	.062	.186	.084	.027	58
Adjusted Predicted Value	4.012	7.013	5.686	.5942	58
Residual	-1.6242	.7479	.0000	.4711	58
Std. Residual	-3.417	1.574	.000	.991	58
Stud. Residual	3.467	1.592	.000	1.007	58
Deleted Residual	-1.6622	.7653	.0005	.4866	58
Stud. Deleted Residual	-3.863	1.614	-.015	1.057	58
Mahal. Distance	.000	7.768	.983	1.515	58
Cook's Distance	.000	.251	.017	.040	58
Centered Leverage Value	.000	.136	.017	.027	58

a. Dependent Variable: HbA1c (%)

Output 2.22 Statistics about the residual

The residuals statistics tell us about the residuals. The mean (SD) for predicted values (HbA1c) is 5.686 (0.5959)%, while HbA1c that we observed is 5.686 (0.7596)%. In a good model, there should be very few residual and our residual here is around 0 ranging from −1.62 to 0.74. The maximum Cook's distance is 0.251, and therefore there is no serious influential point even though previously there was a value (case number 3) that we suspect as an outlier. So we can keep that value in the model.

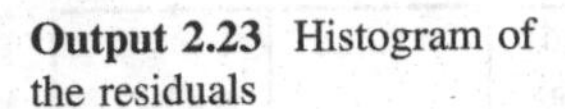
Output 2.23 Histogram of the residuals

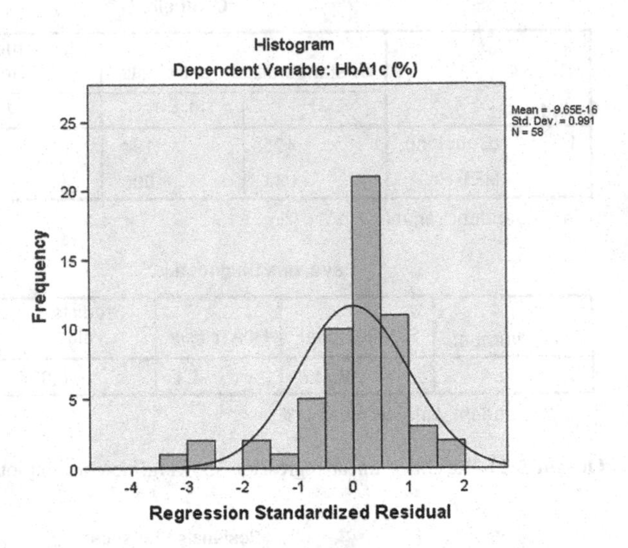

The histogram (Output 2.23) indicates that the residuals are indeed skewed a bit to the left and there is no obvious pattern for residuals and predicted values (Output 2.24). Therefore, we can accept that this regression model is normally distributed.

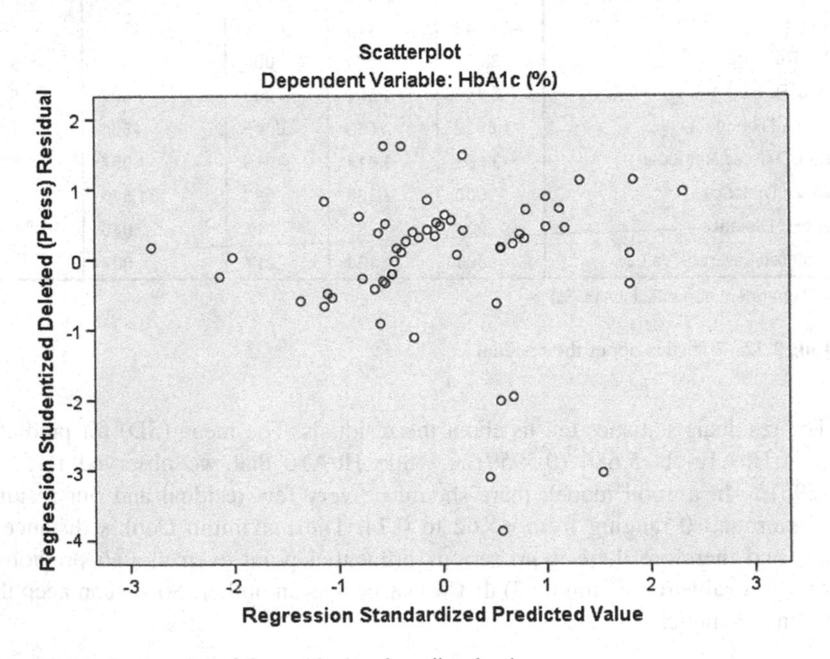

Output 2.24 Scatter plot of the residual and predicted value

Table 2.4 Choosing GLM statistics

Dependant variable	Independent variable	Type of statistics
Single numerical	Single categorical	One-way ANOVA
Single numerical	Multiple categorical	ANOVA
Multiple numerical	Single or multiple numerical	MANOVA
Single numerical	Mixed categorical and numerical	ANCOVA
Multiple numerical	Mixed categorical and numerical	MANCOVA
Repeated numerical	More than two options categorical variable with or without numerical variable (covariate)	Repeated measures ANOVA

ANOVA Analysis of Variance
MANOVA Multiple Analysis of Variance
ANCOVA Analysis of Covariance
MANCOVA Multiple Analysis of Covariance

Using this simple linear regression, physical activity has negative association with diabetic control. If we wish to test whether this conclusion still valid after we take age and BMI into account, we have to do multiple linear regression with age, BMI and MET-Hr as the independent variables. We cannot include sex in linear regression model because sex is a categorical variable. In SPSS we need to use General Linear Model to run such regression.

2.7 General Linear Model

General Linear Model (GLM) is basically a group of statistics that are taking linearity between two sets of measurements as the founding principle. Linearity has been explained in Sect. 2.6 above. In SPSS, to run simple and multiple linear regression, all variables involved must be numerical. GLM could analyse relationship between numerical dependant and categorical independent, or mixed numerical and categorical independent variables. However, the dependant variable should always be numerical, either for single, multiple or repeated measurements (Table 2.4).[13]

[13]Basically, if there are two independent categorical variables, it will be two-way ANOVA, but we do not need to state the number for every analysis. ANOVA should suffice.

A study to determine factors that affecting systolic blood pressure (SBP) among 75 adults. Factor being studied are age (in years), daily calories (0=Within recommended dietary allowance (RDA); 1=Above RDA) and physical activity level (0=Low, 1=Moderate and 2=High).

Data 2.6 Factor affecting systolic blood pressure

2.7.1 ANOVA and ANCOVA

In this section, we will learn how to run ANOVA, specifically two-way ANOVA. One-way ANOVA had been mentioned in Sect. 2.3. Two-way ANOVA means there are two independent variables (or also called as factor). The dependant variable must be in numerical measurement. We can have more than one independent variable but we should not put too many variables into the multivariate model[14] .

Important requirements for ANOVA are as follows:

1. Dependent variable is a numerical measure
2. Distribution of the dependant variable is Normal
3. Variances are homogenous
4. Independent variables are categorical[15]

For this analysis, we will be using Data 2.6, a study on relationship between blood pressure, diet and physical activity.

SPSS Analysis: Univariate GLM

1. Click Analyze
2. Click General Linear Model
3. Click Univariate
4. Move SBP to Dependant Variable box
5. Move Physical activity and Calories intake to Fixed Factors box
6. Click Model
7. Click Custom
8. Change Type to Main effects (assuming no Interaction between independent variables)
9. Move phys and calorie to Model box
10. Click Continue

[14]There are few guidelines about how many independent variables are allowed in one multivariate model. The most common one is 30 samples for each independent factor (VanVoorhis and Morgan 2007). For example, if you have 100 samples, the recommended number of independent variables is 3.

[15]If there is numerical independent variable, it should be called ANCOVA, i.e. Analysis of Co-variance.

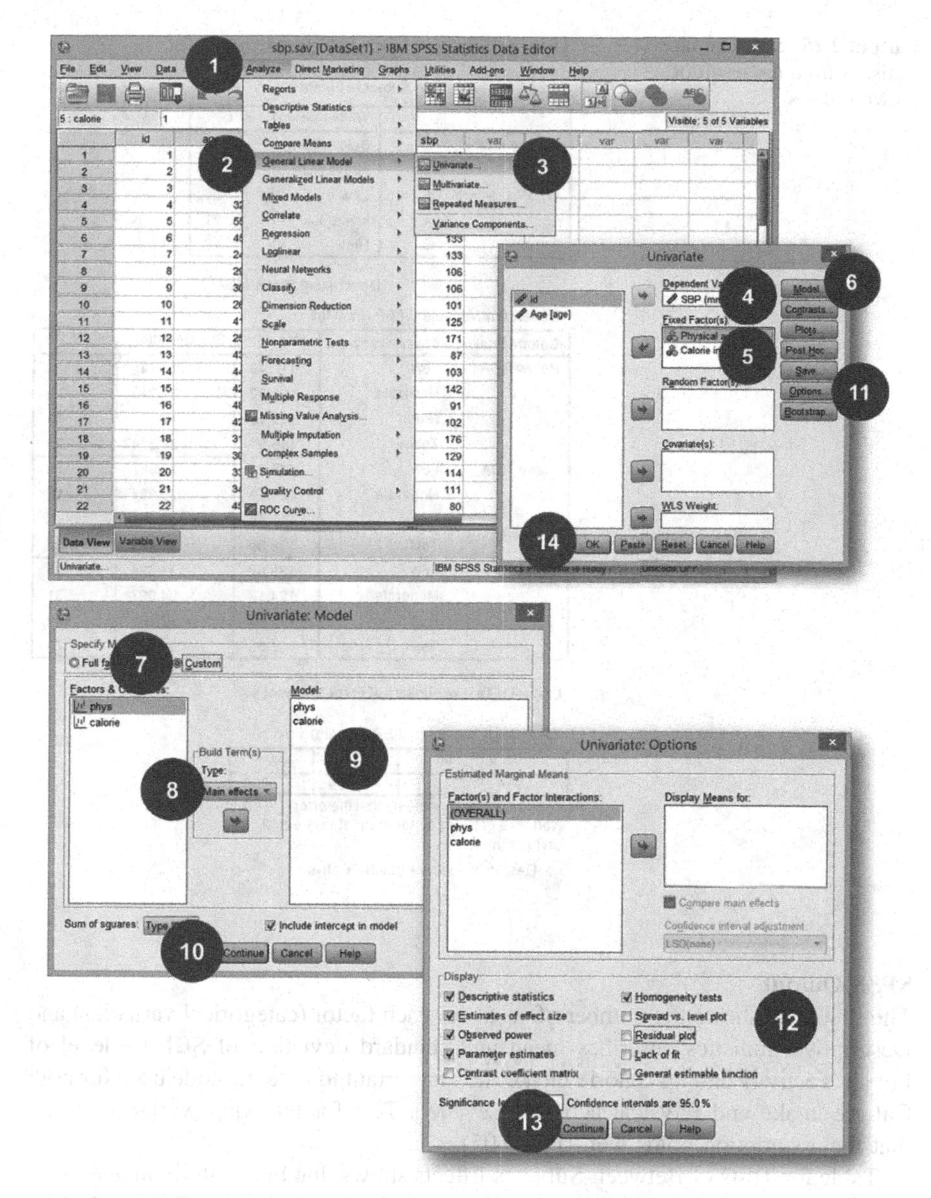

Screen 2.17 How to run linear regression using GLM in SPSS

11. Click Options
12. Check Descriptive statistics, Estimates of effect size, Observed power, Parameter estimates and Homogeneity tests
13. Click Continue
14. Click OK

Output 2.25 Some initial statistics from the result of GLM analysis

Univariate Analysis of Variance

Between-Subjects Factors

		Value Label	N
Calorie intake	0	Below RDA	35
	1	Above RDA	40
Physical activity	0	Low	26
	1	Moderate	31
	2	High	18

Descriptive Statistics

Dependent Variable: SBP (mmHg)

Calorie intake	Physical activity	Mean	Std. Deviation	N
Below RDA	Low	113.43	17.145	7
	Moderate	120.33	27.249	15
	High	112.15	18.685	13
	Total	115.91	22.274	35
Above RDA	Low	149.26	19.067	19
	Moderate	127.69	20.985	16
	High	118.60	12.681	5
	Total	136.80	22.491	40
Total	Low	139.62	24.394	26
	Moderate	124.13	24.097	31
	High	113.94	17.121	18
	Total	127.05	24.588	75

Levene's Test of Equality of Error Variances[a]

Dependent Variable: SBP (mmHg)

F	df1	df2	Sig.
.800	5	69	.553

Tests the null hypothesis that the error variance of the dependent variable is equal across groups.

a. Design: Intercept + calorie + phys

SPSS Output

The first table shows the number of cases for each factor (categorical variables) and Descriptive Statistics describes mean and standard deviation of SBP by level of Physical activity and by Calorie intake. It is important to note the code used for both Calorie intake and Physical activity. Levene's Test for the equal variance shows that the assumption holds well ($P > 0.05$).

Table for Tests of Between-Subjects Effects shows that both calorie intake (diet) and physical activity significantly influence systolic blood pressure ($P < 0.05$). The size of the effect can be seen in the Parameter Estimates[16] table. Taking below the recommended dietary allowance resulted in lower SBP suggested by β of -16.002, while low physical activity increases SBP over 18 mmHg and moderate physical activity increases more than 6 mmHg compared to high physical activity.

[16]In this table, the reference category is the last category.

Tests of Between-Subjects Effects

Dependent Variable: SBP (mmHg)

Source	Type III Sum of Squares	df	Mean Square	F	Sig.	Partial Eta Squared	Noncent. Parameter	Observed Power[b]
Corrected Model	11677.957[a]	3	3892.652	8.359	.000	.261	25.078	.991
Intercept	1126976.195	1	1126976.195	2420.172	.000	.971	2420.172	1.000
calorie	4216.752	1	4216.752	9.055	.004	.113	9.055	.843
phys	3535.313	2	1767.656	3.796	.027	.097	7.592	.674
Error	33061.830	71	465.660					
Total	1255431.000	75						
Corrected Total	44739.787	74						

a. R Squared = .261 (Adjusted R Squared = .230)

b. Computed using alpha = .05

Parameter Estimates

Dependent Variable: SBP (mmHg)

Parameter	B	Std. Error	t	Sig.	95% Confidence Interval Lower Bound	Upper Bound	Partial Eta Squared	Noncent. Parameter	Observed Power[b]
Intercept	125.501	6.373	19.692	.000	112.793	138.209	.845	19.692	1.000
[calorie=0]	-16.002	5.318	-3.009	.004	-26.604	-5.399	.113	3.009	.843
[calorie=1]	0[a]	.	.	.	.	.	.	.	.
[phys=0]	18.422	7.041	2.616	.011	4.382	32.463	.088	2.616	.733
[phys=1]	6.371	6.519	.977	.332	-6.628	19.369	.013	.977	.161
[phys=2]	0[a]	.	.	.	.	.	.	.	.

a. This parameter is set to zero because it is redundant.

b. Computed using alpha = .05

Output 2.26 Tables showing contribution of variables in the model

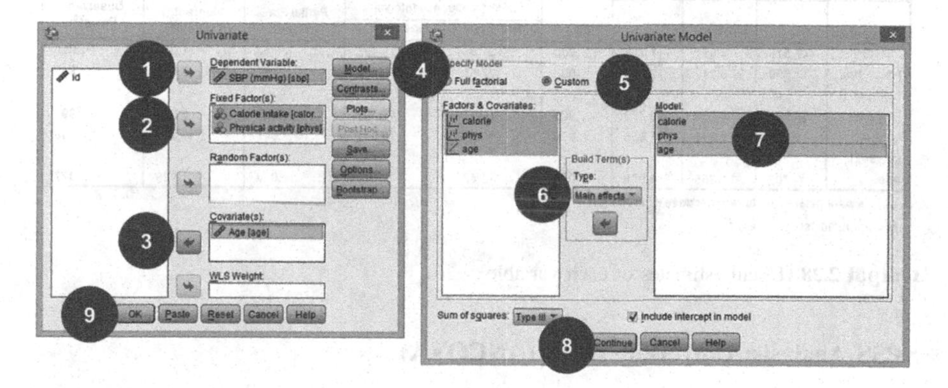

Screen 2.18 ANCOVA in GLM by including numerical variable as covariate

ANOVA in GLM provides Partial Eta Squared (η_p^2) for the effect size and observed power. However, the use of η_p^2 had been discussed elsewhere and must be used with caution (Levine and Hullett 2002; Pierce 2004).

Analysis of covariance (ANCOVA) is quite similar to ANOVA; the different is ANCOVA involves at least a covariate, a numerical variable as one of the independent variables. Using the same Data 2.6 as above, by adding Age as the covariate, we can now use GLM for ANCOVA.

Levene's Test of Equality of Error Variances[a]

Dependent Variable: SBP (mmHg)

F	df1	df2	Sig.
.760	5	69	.582

Tests the null hypothesis that the error variance of the dependent variable is equal across groups.

a. Design: Intercept + calorie + phys + age

Tests of Between-Subjects Effects

Dependent Variable: SBP (mmHg)

Source	Type III Sum of Squares	df	Mean Square	F	Sig.	Partial Eta Squared	Noncent. Parameter	Observed Power[b]
Corrected Model	13347.324[a]	4	3336.831	7.441	.000	.298	29.762	.995
Intercept	53295.736	1	53295.736	118.841	.000	.629	118.841	1.000
calorie	4736.087	1	4736.087	10.561	.002	.131	10.561	.893
phys	5046.061	2	2523.030	5.626	.005	.138	11.252	.845
age	1669.367	1	1669.367	3.722	.058	.050	3.722	.477
Error	31392.463	70	448.464					
Total	1255431.000	75						
Corrected Total	44739.787	74						

a. R Squared = .298 (Adjusted R Squared = .258)

b. Computed using alpha = .05

Output 2.27 Contribution of variables in the model

Parameter Estimates

Dependent Variable: SBP (mmHg)

Parameter	B	Std. Error	t	Sig.	95% Confidence Interval		Partial Eta Squared	Noncent. Parameter	Observed Power[b]
					Lower Bound	Upper Bound			
Intercept	147.513	13.011	11.338	.000	121.564	173.463	.647	11.338	1.000
[calorie=0]	-17.050	5.247	-3.250	.002	-27.514	-6.586	.131	3.250	.893
[calorie=1]	0[a]	.	.	.	.	.	.	.	.
[phys=0]	25.960	7.938	3.270	.002	10.128	41.792	.133	3.270	.897
[phys=1]	13.905	7.495	1.855	.068	-1.044	28.853	.047	1.855	.448
[phys=2]	0[a]	.	.	.	.	.	.	.	.
age	-.703	.365	-1.929	.058	-1.430	.024	.050	1.929	.477

a. This parameter is set to zero because it is redundant.

b. Computed using alpha = .05

Output 2.28 Detail estimates of each variable

SPSS Analysis: Univariate GLM (ANCOVA)

1. Move SBP into Dependent Variable box
2. Move Calorie intake and Physical activity (categorical variables) into Fixed Factors box
3. Move Age into Covariate(s) box
4. Click Model tab
5. Check custom (again assuming to interaction)
6. Choose Main effects as Built Term Type
7. Move all variables into Model box
8. Click Continue
9. Click OK (after you have checked necessary statistics in Options Tab)

SPSS Output
The first two tables from the analysis are the same like ANOVA. Levene's test again shows that the assumption for equal variances still valid (P > 0.05). ANCOVA shows that Age is not associated with SBP (P = 0.058) when controlled for Calorie intake and Physical activity. Calorie intake and physical activity are still significantly associated with SBP (P = 0.02 and P = 0.05, respectively).

2.7.2 *MANOVA and MANCOVA*

The letter 'M' means multiple dependent variables. Just like ANOVA and ANCOVA, the difference between Multivariate ANOVA (MANOVA) or Multivariate ANCOVA (MANCOVA) is the presence of numerical variables as independent variables.

To illustrate MANOVA, we will use Data 2.7, a study on the use of biomaterial for bone loss in fracture.

The outcomes of interest are total hospital cost (in $) and length of stay (LOS, measured in days). The main factor under study is type of bone graft used (either patient's own bone, Autograft, or a bone substitute, labelled as Biomaterial). The main confounder to Cost and LOS is the fracture's site because different bones require different times to unite. Age was recorded as another possible confounder because young patient heals faster. Our aim is to show the efficacy of bone substitutes compared to autograft.

> Bone lost during fracture is common. The gold standard to manage bone lost is using autologous bone graft harvested usually from iliac crest to fill in the gap. Recently there are already many new biomaterial that can substitute or can be used in conjunction with patient's own bone graft. Some studies showed that the combination of biomaterial with platelet can increase efficacy. A trial was conducted among 80 patients who sustained fracture of long bones (humerus, tibia or femur) to compare the effectiveness of this biomaterial and biomaterial plus platelet versus autograft. The outcome measured was the total hospital cost ($) and the length of stay (days). Age of patients was recorded as a possible confounder apart from the site of fracture mentioned above.

Data 2.7 Biomaterial versus autograft in fractured long bone

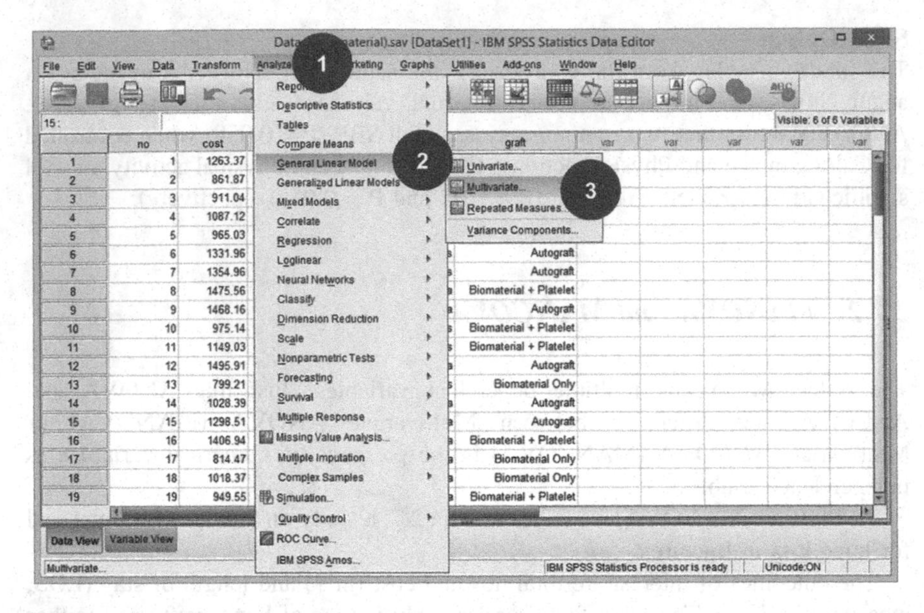

Screen 2.19 How to run Multivariate GLM

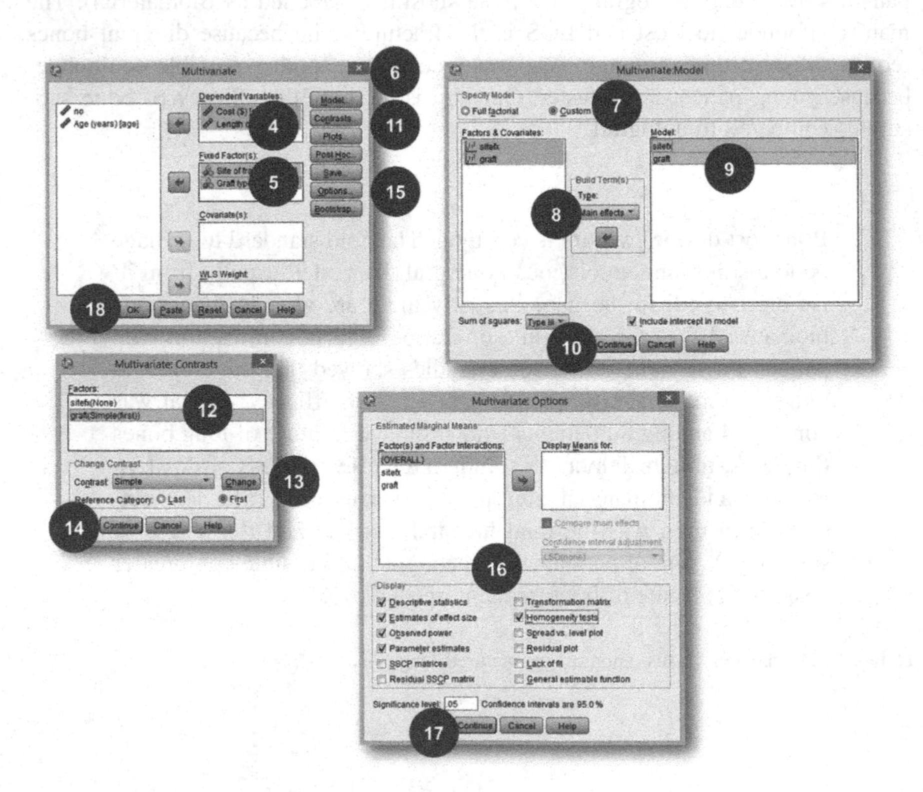

Screen 2.20 How to run Multivariate GLM

Between-Subjects Factors

		Value Label	N
Site of fracture	0	Humerus	39
	1	Tibia	34
	2	Femur	7
Graft type	0	Autograft	29
	1	Biomaterial + Platelet	27
	2	Biomaterial Only	24

Descriptive Statistics

	Site of fracture	Graft type	Mean	Std. Deviation	N
Cost ($)	Humerus	Autograft	1267.9040	91.21309	15
		Biomaterial + Platelet	1089.6687	164.32559	15
		Biomaterial Only	1001.2367	224.42255	9
		Total	1137.8133	188.75932	39
	Tibia	Autograft	1405.5377	192.04612	13
		Biomaterial + Platelet	1195.6856	210.78838	9
		Biomaterial Only	999.8992	155.76268	12
		Total	1206.8221	251.85256	34
	Femur	Autograft	1002.8100	.	1
		Biomaterial + Platelet	1130.7400	320.19216	3
		Biomaterial Only	1192.2400	201.85971	3
		Total	1138.8214	228.69062	7
	Total	Autograft	1320.4607	168.55356	29
		Biomaterial + Platelet	1129.5711	196.28941	27
		Biomaterial Only	1024.4433	191.99680	24
		Total	1167.2302	220.86177	80
Length of stay (days)	Humerus	Autograft	7.960	1.0682	15
		Biomaterial + Platelet	9.120	1.2055	15
		Biomaterial Only	8.689	1.0717	9
		Total	8.574	1.2113	39
	Tibia	Autograft	8.462	.8242	13
		Biomaterial + Platelet	9.100	1.3238	9
		Biomaterial Only	9.483	1.0650	12
		Total	8.991	1.1188	34
	Femur	Autograft	10.900	.	1
		Biomaterial + Platelet	10.133	1.6503	3
		Biomaterial Only	10.267	2.9195	3
		Total	10.300	1.9553	7
	Total	Autograft	8.286	1.0849	29
		Biomaterial + Platelet	9.226	1.2799	27
		Biomaterial Only	9.283	1.4030	24
		Total	8.903	1.3223	80

Output 2.29 Descriptive output from Multivariate GLM

Box's Test of Equality of Covariance Matrices[a]

Box's M	55.648
F	2.159
df1	21
df2	841.799
Sig.	.002

Tests the null hypothesis that the observed covariance matrices of the dependent variables are equal across groups.

a. Design: Intercept + sitefx + graft

Levene's Test of Equality of Error Variances[a]

	F	df1	df2	Sig.
Cost ($)	2.023	8	71	.056
Length of stay (days)	1.928	8	71	.069

Tests the null hypothesis that the error variance of the dependent variable is equal across groups.

a. Design: Intercept + sitefx + graft

Output 2.30 Diagnostic test results

SPSS Analysis: Multivariate GLM

1. Click Analyse
2. Click General Linear Model
3. Click Multivariate
4. Move Cost and Length of stay into Dependant Variables box
5. Move Site of fracture and Graft type into Fixed Factor(s) box
6. Click Model
7. Check Custom
8. Change Build Term type to Main effects (assuming no interaction)
9. Move both variables into Model box
10. Click Continue (go back to Multivariate box)
11. Click Contrasts[17]
12. Click on graft (to assign reference point)
13. Choose Simple as contrast method and check First (assigning Autograft as the reference category)
14. Click Continue (go back to Multivariate box)
15. Click Options
16. Check Descriptive statistics, Estimates of effect size, Observed power, Parameter estimates and Homogeneity tests
17. Click Continue (go back to Multivariate box)
18. Click OK

[17]This is an important step to understand the result based on our objective to describe the relationship between type of material used and both dependent variables.

Multivariate Tests[a]

Effect		Value	F	Hypothesis df	Error df	Sig.	Partial Eta Squared	Noncent. Parameter	Observed Power[d]
Intercept	Pillai's Trace	.990	3816.451[b]	2.000	74.000	.000	.990	7632.903	1.000
	Wilks' Lambda	.010	3816.451[b]	2.000	74.000	.000	.990	7632.903	1.000
	Hotelling's Trace	103.147	3816.451[b]	2.000	74.000	.000	.990	7632.903	1.000
	Roy's Largest Root	103.147	3816.451[b]	2.000	74.000	.000	.990	7632.903	1.000
sitefx	Pillai's Trace	.222	4.694	4.000	150.000	.001	.111	18.774	.945
	Wilks' Lambda	.781	4.859[b]	4.000	148.000	.001	.116	19.435	.953
	Hotelling's Trace	.275	5.019	4.000	146.000	.001	.121	20.076	.959
	Roy's Largest Root	.256	9.601[c]	2.000	75.000	.000	.204	19.201	.977
graft	Pillai's Trace	.357	8.138	4.000	150.000	.000	.178	32.551	.998
	Wilks' Lambda	.651	8.841[b]	4.000	148.000	.000	.193	35.363	.999
	Hotelling's Trace	.523	9.536	4.000	146.000	.000	.207	38.145	1.000
	Roy's Largest Root	.498	18.658[c]	2.000	75.000	.000	.332	37.315	1.000

a. Design: Intercept + sitefx + graft

b. Exact statistic

c. The statistic is an upper bound on F that yields a lower bound on the significance level.

d. Computed using alpha = .05

Output 2.31 Multivariate tests table

Tests of Between-Subjects Effects

Source	Dependent Variable	Type III Sum of Squares	df	Mean Square	F	Sig.	Partial Eta Squared	Noncent. Parameter	Observed Power[c]
Corrected Model	Cost ($)	1340031.61[a]	4	335007.903	9.996	.000	.348	39.984	1.000
	Length of stay (days)	31.414[b]	4	7.853	5.519	.001	.227	22.076	.970
Intercept	Cost ($)	61796368.11	1	61796368.11	1843.874	.000	.961	1843.874	1.000
	Length of stay (days)	3891.225	1	3891.225	2734.502	.000	.973	2734.502	1.000
sitefx	Cost ($)	131517.974	2	65758.987	1.962	.148	.050	3.924	.394
	Length of stay (days)	14.094	2	7.047	4.952	.010	.117	9.904	.795
graft	Cost ($)	1247337.954	2	623668.977	18.609	.000	.332	37.218	1.000
	Length of stay (days)	13.276	2	6.638	4.665	.012	.111	9.329	.769
Error	Cost ($)	2513582.061	75	33514.427					
	Length of stay (days)	106.726	75	1.423					
Total	Cost ($)	112847730.2	80						
	Length of stay (days)	6478.500	80						
Corrected Total	Cost ($)	3853613.672	79						
	Length of stay (days)	138.139	79						

a. R Squared = .348 (Adjusted R Squared = .313)

b. R Squared = .227 (Adjusted R Squared = .186)

c. Computed using alpha = .05

Parameter Estimates

Dependent Variable	Parameter	B	Std. Error	t	Sig.	95% Confidence Interval		Partial Eta Squared	Noncent. Parameter	Observed Power[b]
						Lower Bound	Upper Bound			
Cost ($)	Intercept	1043.530	74.241	14.056	.000	895.634	1191.426	.725	14.056	1.000
	[sitefx=0]	-69.874	75.991	-.920	.361	-221.255	81.507	.011	.920	.148
	[sitefx=1]	14.232	76.702	.186	.853	-138.566	167.030	.000	.186	.054
	[sitefx=2]	0[a]	.	.	.	.	.	.	.	.
	[graft=0]	306.692	51.115	6.000	.000	204.866	408.519	.324	6.000	1.000
	[graft=1]	120.116	51.916	2.314	.023	16.694	223.538	.067	2.314	.627
	[graft=2]	0[a]	.	.	.	.	.	.	.	.
Length of stay (days)	Intercept	10.405	.484	21.509	.000	9.442	11.369	.861	21.509	1.000
	[sitefx=0]	-1.522	.495	-3.073	.003	-2.508	-.535	.112	3.073	.858
	[sitefx=1]	-1.103	.500	-2.206	.030	-2.098	-.107	.061	2.206	.586
	[sitefx=2]	0[a]	.	.	.	.	.	.	.	.
	[graft=0]	-.838	.333	-2.515	.014	-1.501	-.174	.078	2.515	.699
	[graft=1]	.034	.338	.099	.921	-.640	.707	.000	.099	.051
	[graft=2]	0[a]	.	.	.	.	.	.	.	.

a. This parameter is set to zero because it is redundant.

b. Computed using alpha = .05

Output 2.32 Between subject test and parameter estimates

Contrast Results (K Matrix)

Graft type Simple Contrast[a]			Dependent Variable: Cost ($)	Dependent Variable: Length of stay (days)
Level 2 vs. Level 1	Contrast Estimate		-176.998	.871
	Hypothesized Value		0	0
	Difference (Estimate - Hypothesized)		-176.998	.871
	Std. Error		50.362	.322
	Sig.		.001	.008
	95% Confidence Interval for Difference	Lower Bound	-277.325	.230
		Upper Bound	-76.671	1.512
Level 3 vs. Level 1	Contrast Estimate		-307.077	.838
	Hypothesized Value		0	0
	Difference (Estimate - Hypothesized)		-307.077	.838
	Std. Error		52.114	.333
	Sig.		.000	.014
	95% Confidence Interval for Difference	Lower Bound	-410.893	.174
		Upper Bound	-203.261	1.501

a. Reference category = 1

Output 2.33 Custom contrast result

SPSS Output

The first table shows the value label and the count for each category option. Second table shows descriptive statistics for both outcomes. Overall, Autograft cost the highest ($1320) and Biomaterial only is the cheapest ($1024). Those treated with autograft discharged earliest (8.3 days) than those treated with biomaterial alone or biomaterial with platelet (9.3 and 9.2 days, respectively).

Both Box's test and Levene's test homogeneity. Box's M test equals of variance multivariate, whilst Levene's test equals variance for each dependent variables. Box's M test shows that the variance cannot be assumed as equal multivariate but since Box's M test is known to be very sensitive to deviation from normal distribution, its result carry little effect to the analysis. In this analysis, Levene's test shows that variance for both Cost and LOS are equal ($P > 0.05$).

The Multivariate Tests table (Output 2.31) shows the effect of each independent variable (and their interaction if included in the model) towards overall dependent variables. This table shows that type of graft and fracture site have statistically significant relationship with both outcomes. However, this table does not provide information that we really want, i.e. which graft is the best.

Test of Between-Subjects Effects and Parameter Estimates provide detailed effect of each independent variable to different outcomes. In Parameter Estimates, we cannot change the reference point. By default, the last category will become the reference point. For example, graft = 2 or Biomaterial Only is the reference point. So Autograft and Biomaterial with Platelet will be compared to Biomaterial Only.

Since our aim is to compare grafts with autograft, it would be better if we set autograft as the reference point. For that matter, we should use Contrast.

The next, and in fact the most useful table, is the Contrast Results (the result for Step #11–13). In this table, Level 2 (Biomaterial with Platelet) is compared to Level 1 (Autograft). The analysis shows that the cost was significantly lowered by $177 but length of stay in the hospital significantly increased to 0.9 day. Biomaterial only further lowers the cost up to $308 and increased hospital stay to 0.8 day.

The analysis shows that using the grafts we may be able to cut the cost but patient will heal slower.

Site of fracture is not discussed here because this is a known fact that site of fracture is indeed affecting healing process and hence affecting length of stay, and therefore the cost too.

MANCOVA is done if we include age as the covariate. The discussion of outcomes is the same.

2.7.3 *Repeated Measures ANOVA*

Repeated measures basically means observing same variable repeatedly. We might be interested to repeat blood glucose test of same diabetic patients who come to our clinic every month to measure how effective our treatment is, or we might be interested to monitor fitness level of some similar athletes taking special exercise and diet programme over regular intervals. Since we are measuring blood glucose of the same patients over times or fitness level of the same athletes over times,

	Low	Fasting Blood Sugar (mmol/L)			
Patient	**Sugar Diet**	**Day 1**	**Day 2**	**Day 3**	**Day 4**
A	No	13.2	12.1	11.3	9.7
B	No	13.4	11.3	10.2	9.2
C	No	12.9	10.3	9.8	8.6
D	No	11.9	10.6	9.7	8.9
E	No	10.6	9.6	8.3	6.1
F	Yes	12.3	11.1	8.3	6.4
G	Yes	12.1	10.5	7.6	6.5
H	Yes	13.4	9.8	7.2	5.9
I	Yes	12.6	9.6	7.4	5.5
J	Yes	12.9	9.5	8.1	6.2

Data 2.8 Blood sugar control

the measurements are related. Their second measurement is affected both by our treatment and by the previous value.

How could we summarise repeated measures? We can compare the means differences over time, compare the maximum (or minimum) values, compare area under the curve or compare the rate of change. In this book, we will be using ANOVA to describe and to test the differences over different groups. In one-way ANOVA where there is only one numerical dependent variable and one categorical independent variable, we test between-groups variances. In one-way repeated measures ANOVA with multiple (i.e. more than two) related dependent variables, we need to test within-groups variances as well.

Let us take the example as displayed in Data 2.8. This is a study to measure the effect of low sugar diet in managing diabetic patients. All patients have comparable sex and age, received same medication and had their fasting blood sugar measured daily for 4 days. The patients are divided in two groups: those receive low sugar diet and those do not.

Assumptions used in SPSS for repeated measures ANOVA are as follows:

1. All dependent variables have multivariate normal distribution
2. The covariance matrix of dependent variables is constant across all independent variables (when P > 0.10 in Box's Test)
3. Covariance matrix of the dependent variables is spherical (sphericity assumption) (Mauchly's Test of Sphericity P > 0.05 confirm the assumption)

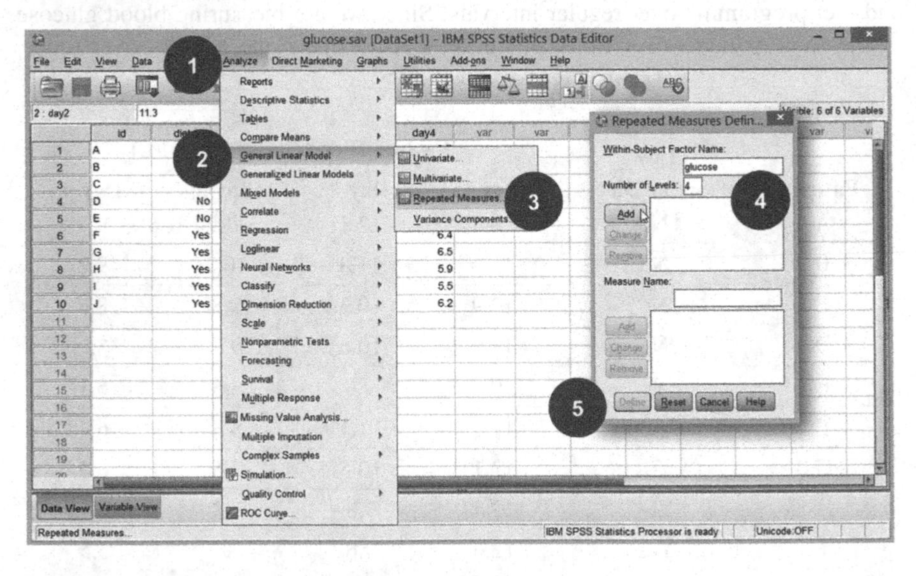

Screen 2.21 How to run Repeated Measures ANOVA

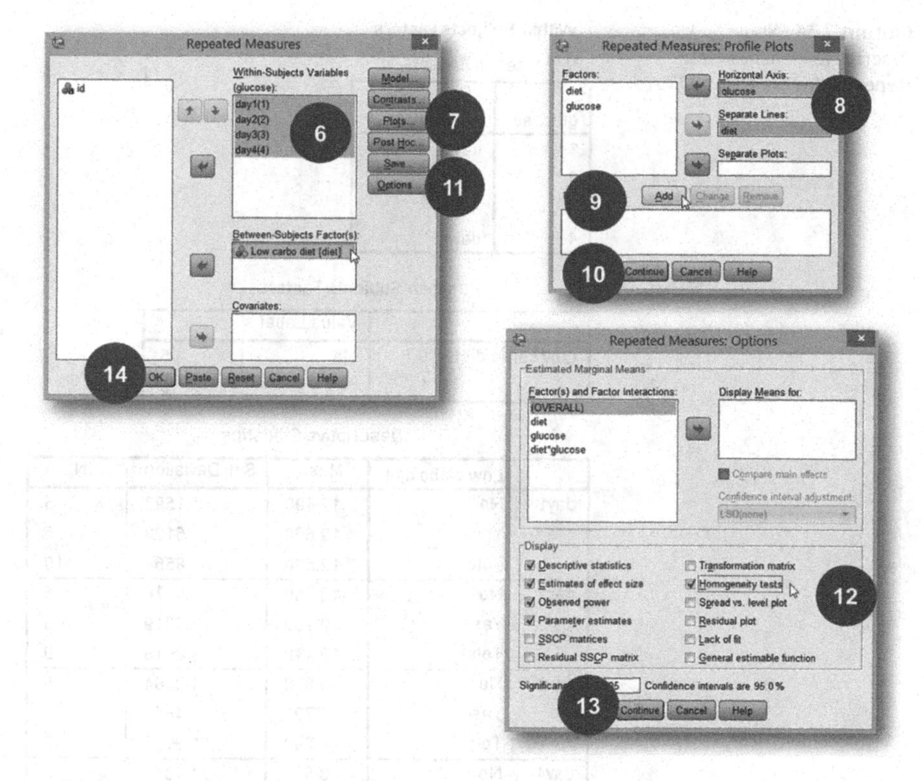

Screen 2.22 How to run Repeated Measures ANOVA

SPSS Analysis: Repeated Measures ANOVA

1. Click Analyze
2. Click General Linear Model
3. Click Repeated Measures
4. Type glucose (or any label you prefer) in Within-Subject Factor Name box. Type 4 into Number of Levels box (because we have 4 repeated measurements of blood glucose). Click Add.
5. Click Define
6. Move all 4 days (day1, day2, day3 and day4) into Within-Subjects Variables box. Careful with the order. Move Low carbo diet into Between-Subject Factor (s) box
7. Click Plots
8. Move glucose into Horizontal Axis and diet into Separate Lines box
9. Click Add

Output 2.34 Some descriptive statistics from Repeated Measures ANOVA

Within-Subjects Factors

Measure: MEASURE_1

glucose	Dependent Variable
1	day1
2	day2
3	day3
4	day4

Between-Subjects Factors

		Value Label	N
Low carbo diet	0	No	5
	1	Yes	5

Descriptive Statistics

	Low carbo diet	Mean	Std. Deviation	N
day1	No	12.400	1.1597	5
	Yes	12.660	.5128	5
	Total	12.530	.8564	10
day2	No	10.780	.9576	5
	Yes	10.100	.6819	5
	Total	10.440	.8618	10
day3	No	9.860	1.0784	5
	Yes	7.720	.4658	5
	Total	8.790	1.3731	10
day4	No	8.500	1.4018	5
	Yes	6.100	.4062	5
	Total	7.300	1.5958	10

10. Click Continue
11. Click Options
12. Check Descriptive statistics, Estimates of effect sizes, Observed power, Parameter estimates and Homogeneity tests
13. Click Continue
14. Click OK

SPSS Output

The first three tables describe dependent variable, independent variable and the overall description. We can observe that the average blood glucose decreased from 12.5 to 7.3 mmol/L (total for each day). Those taking low carbohydrate diet had better blood glucose reduction (12.7–6.1 mmol/L) compared to those not taking the special diet (12.4–8.5 mmol/L).

There are many more tables in the output, but the next important output to look at first is the Profile Plot.

Output 2.35 The profile plot

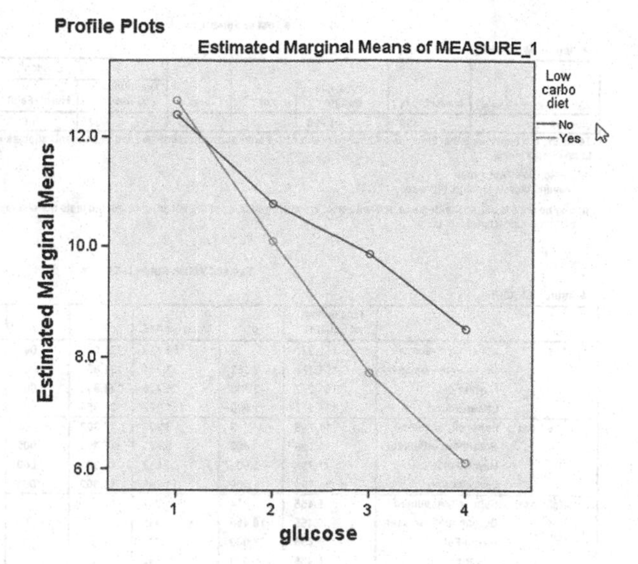

Box's Test of Equality of Covariance Matrices[a]

Box's M	13.377
F	.575
df1	10
df2	305.976
Sig.	.834

Tests the null hypothesis that the observed covariance matrices of the dependent variables are equal across groups.

a. Design: Intercept + diet
Within Subjects Design: glucose

Multivariate Tests[a]

Effect		Value	F	Hypothesis df	Error df	Sig.	Partial Eta Squared	Noncent. Parameter	Observed Power[c]
glucose	Pillai's Trace	.990	202.317[b]	3.000	6.000	.000	.990	606.951	1.000
	Wilks' Lambda	.010	202.317[b]	3.000	6.000	.000	.990	606.951	1.000
	Hotelling's Trace	101.159	202.317[b]	3.000	6.000	.000	.990	606.951	1.000
	Roy's Largest Root	101.159	202.317[b]	3.000	6.000	.000	.990	606.951	1.000
glucose * diet	Pillai's Trace	.903	18.577[b]	3.000	6.000	.002	.903	55.732	.996
	Wilks' Lambda	.097	18.577[b]	3.000	6.000	.002	.903	55.732	.996
	Hotelling's Trace	9.289	18.577[b]	3.000	6.000	.002	.903	55.732	.996
	Roy's Largest Root	9.289	18.577[b]	3.000	6.000	.002	.903	55.732	.996

a. Design: Intercept + diet
Within Subjects Design: glucose

b. Exact statistic

c. Computed using alpha = .05

Output 2.36 Output from Repeated Measures ANOVA

Mauchly's Test of Sphericity[a]

Measure: MEASURE_1

Within Subjects Effect	Mauchly's W	Approx. Chi-Square	df	Sig.	Epsilon[b] Greenhouse-Geisser	Huynh-Feldt	Lower-bound
glucose	.490	4.796	5	.445	.687	1.000	.333

Tests the null hypothesis that the error covariance matrix of the orthonormalized transformed dependent variables is proportional to an identity matrix.

a. Design: Intercept + diet
Within Subjects Design: glucose

b. May be used to adjust the degrees of freedom for the averaged tests of significance. Corrected tests are displayed in the Tests of Within-Subjects Effects table.

Tests of Within-Subjects Effects

Measure: MEASURE_1

Source		Type III Sum of Squares	df	Mean Square	F	Sig.	Partial Eta Squared	Noncent. Parameter	Observed Power[a]
glucose	Sphericity Assumed	151.277	3	50.426	221.854	.000	.965	665.563	1.000
	Greenhouse-Geisser	151.277	2.062	73.354	221.854	.000	.965	457.528	1.000
	Huynh-Feldt	151.277	3.000	50.426	221.854	.000	.965	665.563	1.000
	Lower-bound	151.277	1.000	151.277	221.854	.000	.965	221.854	1.000
glucose * diet	Sphericity Assumed	11.798	3	3.933	17.302	.000	.684	51.907	1.000
	Greenhouse-Geisser	11.798	2.062	5.721	17.302	.000	.684	35.682	.999
	Huynh-Feldt	11.798	3.000	3.933	17.302	.000	.684	51.907	1.000
	Lower-bound	11.798	1.000	11.798	17.302	.003	.684	17.302	.952
Error(glucose)	Sphericity Assumed	5.455	24	.227					
	Greenhouse-Geisser	5.455	16.498	.331					
	Huynh-Feldt	5.455	24.000	.227					
	Lower-bound	5.455	8.000	.682					

a. Computed using alpha = .05

Output 2.37 Output from Repeated Measures ANOVA

The profile plot above shows the overall within and between changes of the blood glucose.[18] This profile plot illustrates the descriptive table above even better. We could see that overall, the blood glucose decreased over times for both patients with or without special diet but it is more obvious among those with low carbohydrate diet (green line). So are the changes we observed significant statistically?

SPSS repeated measures ANOVA also provides multivariate test. However, multivariate test is rarely used unless there is a severe violation of Sphericity Test. Before we could interpret multivariate test, we need to check the assumption for equality of variances for dependent variables across the factor (Box's Test).

Box's test determines whether there was constant variance of serially measured blood glucoses across different types of diet (multivariate). Since the $P > 0.10$, the assumption is met. The subsequent multivariate tests become valid. SPSS offers four different tests and Pillai's Trace is considered a robust and recommended test (Olson 1974). The statistics shows that there is a significant effect of glucose over times.

The subsequent tables are more relevant for repeated measures.

As mentioned above, we would like to determine both within-subjects and between-subjects effects. First, we check Mauchly's Test for sphericity. In the table above, $P = 0.445$ and therefore the assumption is met. We could then observe the first row for each model. Within-subjects effect for glucose over four different times has **at least one** significant difference ($F(3, 24) = 221.854$, $P < 0.001$, $\eta_p^2 = 0.965$).

[18]If we have more than one independent variable (or factor) and we would like to compare the changes over different plots, make sure that the x-axis scale is comparable. This can be done in Chart editor.

Tests of Between-Subjects Effects

Measure: MEASURE_1
Transformed Variable: Average

Source	Type III Sum of Squares	df	Mean Square	F	Sig.	Partial Eta Squared	Noncent. Parameter	Observed Power[a]
Intercept	3814.209	1	3814.209	1485.212	.000	.995	1485.212	1.000
diet	15.376	1	15.376	5.987	.040	.428	5.987	.575
Error	20.545	8	2.568					

a. Computed using alpha = .05

Output 2.38 Output from Repeated Measures ANOVA

The glucose*diet shows the interaction of glucose and diet over times. If the interaction is significant, it means that the rate of changes for glucose over time between those taking low carbohydrate diet and those not taking the special diet is different. In this analysis, different diets provide different within-subject effects for glucose as well ($F(3, 24) = 17.302$, $P < 0.001$, $\eta_p^2 = 0.684$). The effect of diet can be further confirmed looking at between-subjects effect table.

The ANOVA table shows that the effect of diet on glucose over times is significant ($F(1,8) = 5.987$, $P = 0.040$, $\eta_p^2 = 0.428$). So if our main question when we analyse these data is whether different diets provide different glucose reductions over times, the answer is yes.

In summary, in SPSS, we would want to summarise three important values: (1) univariate within-subject effect of the dependent variables over time; (2) univariate within-subject effect interaction between dependent variable and factor over times and (3) between-subject effect. If all three F tests are significant, we can conclude that there is at least one significant within-subject effect and at least one significant between-subjects effect.

2.8 Logistic Regression

Logistic regression is used when the dependent variable is categorical. The independent variable can be numerical or categorical. In binary logistic regression which is the most popular version of logistic regression, the dependent variable is dichotomous, e.g. dead or alive, disease or health, etc. This book will cover only binomial logistic regression. To illustrate binary logistic regression, we will use Data 2.9.

> A cross sectional study was done in one primary school involving 109 students aged 7-12 years old. All students undergone polysomnography (sleep study) to detect the presence of obstructive sleep apnoea (OSA) coded 0=No, 1=Yes. Other variables include age (in years), gender (0=Female, 1=Male) and BMI status (categorised into 0=Normal, 1=Overweight and 2=Obese based on BMI for age).

Data 2.9 Obstructive sleep apnoea

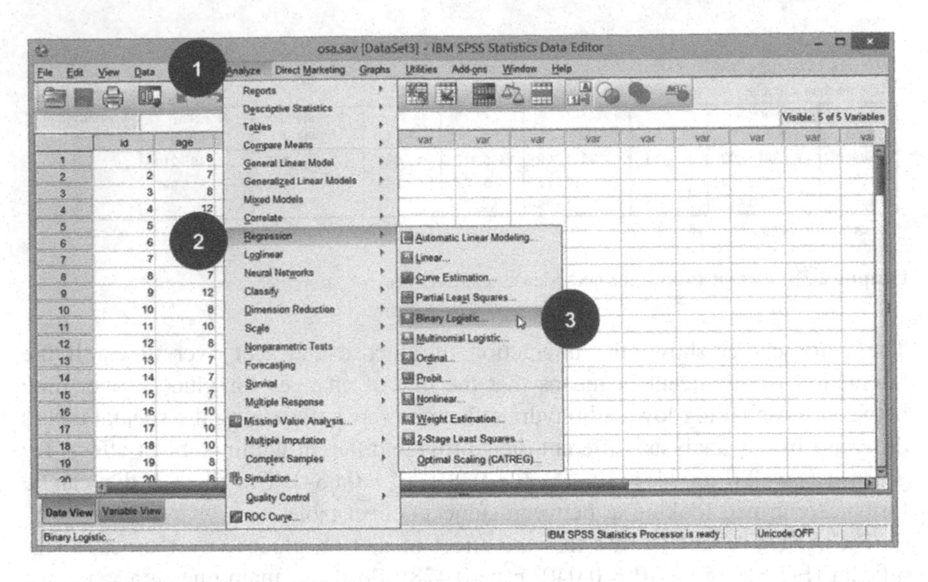

Screen 2.23 How to run Logistic Regression

The aim of the study is determine the relationship of age, gender and BMI with OSA.

SPSS Analysis: Binary logistic regression

1. Click Analyse
2. Click Regression
3. Click Binary
4. Move Obstructive sleep apnoea (osa) to Dependent box[19]
5. Move all independent variables into Covariates box.[20] Leave the Method as Enter.
6. Click Categorical button
7. Move only categorical variables, i.e. Gender and BMI into Categorical Covariates box
8. Change the contrast for both variables to First. Leave the Contrast type as Indicator, keeping the default (First) as the reference point, and click Change
9. Click Continue
10. Click Option button

[19]Make sure that the response code is created with the last option for the factor of interest. In this example, 0 is the response code for No OSA and 1 for Yes OSA. Between 0 and 1, 1 is the last value. If you use 1 and 2, 2 is the last value. So make sure that the last value is the response of your interest. We are interested to measure relationship for OSA, not for those not having OSA. Hence, Yes OSA should be the response of interest.

[20]Even though both Gender and BMI are not numerical values, they are moved into this box but later we will specify which ones are categorical.

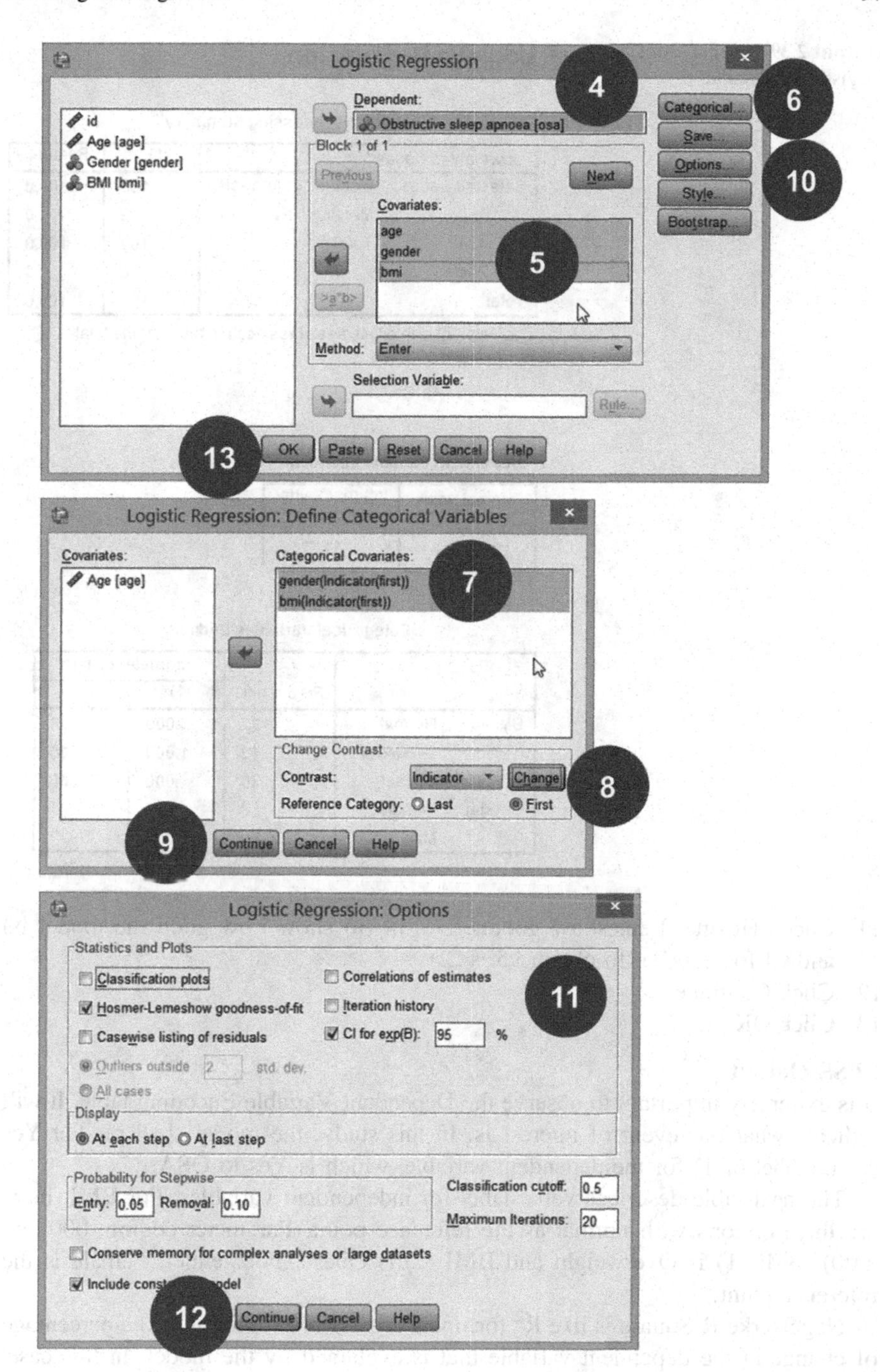

Screen 2.24 How to run Logistic Regression

Output 2.39 Output from Logistic Regression

Logistic Regression

Case Processing Summary

Unweighted Cases[a]		N	Percent
Selected Cases	Included in Analysis	109	100.0
	Missing Cases	0	.0
	Total	109	100.0
Unselected Cases		0	.0
Total		109	100.0

a. If weight is in effect, see classification table for the total number of cases.

Dependent Variable Encoding

Original Value	Internal Value
No	0
Yes	1

Categorical Variables Codings

		Frequency	Parameter coding (1)	(2)
BMI	Normal	37	.000	.000
	Overweight	42	1.000	.000
	Obese	30	.000	1.000
Gender	Female	58	.000	
	Male	51	1.000	

11. Check Hosmer-Lemeshow goodness-of-fit (to show how good the model is) and CI for exp(B) (to obtain 95 %CI)
12. Click Continue
13. Click OK

SPSS Output

It is extremely important to observe the Dependent Variable Encoding table. It will indicate what our event of interest is. In this study, the model shall predict Yes (value label of 1) for the dependent variable, which is Yes to OSA.

The next table describes value label for independent variables. For BMI, there are three options with normal as the reference point (Parameter coding .000 and .000). BMI (1) is Overweight and BMI (2) is Obese. For gender, Female is the reference point.

Nagelkerke R Square is like R^2 for linear regression. It measures the percentage of change in the dependent variable that is explained by the model. In this case, BMI and gender explain 26.8 % changes in OSA. However, the value is not as

Model Summary

Step	-2 Log likelihood	Cox & Snell R Square	Nagelkerke R Square
1	124.225[a]	.199	.268

a. Estimation terminated at iteration number 5 because parameter estimates changed by less than .001.

Hosmer and Lemeshow Test

Step	Chi-square	df	Sig.
1	3.422	7	.843

Output 2.40 Output from Logistic Regression

Contingency Table for Hosmer and Lemeshow Test

		Obstructive sleep apnoea = No		Obstructive sleep apnoea = Yes		Total
		Observed	Expected	Observed	Expected	
Step 1	1	13	12.602	1	1.398	14
	2	8	8.683	2	1.317	10
	3	9	8.821	3	3.179	12
	4	7	7.428	4	3.572	11
	5	9	8.253	5	5.747	14
	6	5	3.556	2	3.444	7
	7	2	3.744	7	5.256	9
	8	5	5.246	9	8.754	14
	9	5	4.667	13	13.333	18

Classification Table[a]

Observed			Predicted: Obstructive sleep apnoea No	Yes	Percentage Correct
Step 1	Obstructive sleep apnoea	No	50	13	79.4
		Yes	16	30	65.2
	Overall Percentage				73.4

a. The cut value is .500

Output 2.41 Output from Logistic Regression

impressive as when we use R^2 in linear regression. So do not take it seriously. More important is Hosmer and Lemeshow's (H-L) test. The test checks whether the model fits. H_o for H-L test is that there is no difference between predicted and observed values. Since the P = 0.843, we could not reject the H_o; therefore, the

Variables in the Equation

		B	S.E.	Wald	df	Sig.	Exp(B)	95% C.I.for EXP(B)	
								Lower	Upper
Step 1[a]	age	.217	.145	2.262	1	.133	1.243	.936	1.650
	gender(1)	1.263	.447	7.973	1	.005	3.535	1.471	8.492
	bmi			6.419	2	.040			
	bmi(1)	1.275	.548	5.418	1	.020	3.579	1.223	10.473
	bmi(2)	1.319	.603	4.778	1	.029	3.738	1.146	12.192
	Constant	-3.721	1.339	7.717	1	.005	.024		

a. Variable(s) entered on step 1: age, gender, bmi.

Output 2.42 Output from Logistic Regression

Table 2.5 Example of logistic regression table

	B	SE	Wald	df	P	OR	95 %CI	
Age	0.217	0.145	2.262	1	0.133	1.24	0.94	1.65
Male[1]	1.263	0.447	7.973	1	0.005	3.53	1.47	8.49
BMI	1.275	0.548	6.419	2	0.040	3.58	1.22	10.47
Overweight[2]	1.319	0.603	5.418	1	0.020	3.74	1.15	12.19
Obese[2]			4.778	1	0.029			

[1]Compared to Female, [2]compared to Normal BMI

observed and predicted values using this logistic regression model are the same, which is what we want. The difference between predicted values from the model versus the observed values (from our data collection) are further described in the next two tables.

Classification table shows that the degree percentage of agreement between predicted and observed values is 73.4 %.

Once the model's fit has been determined, we can describe the main table for logistic regression which is Variables in the Equation table. This table shows that gender and BMI are significant factors associated with OSA ($P = 0.005$ and $P = 0.040$, respectively). Age is not associated with OSA ($P = 0.133$). The result can be summarised as given Table 2.5.

2.9 How to Analyse, in Summary

1. Make sure we have a very clear general objective and more importantly detail specific objectives
2. For every specific objective, identify the variable involved and their level of measurement
3. Decide what we want. Whether we want to describe certain variables, or we may want to test the association. However, always remember that cross-sectional study does not able to prove any causation because of the lack of temporal association.

4. The statistics we use depends on what we want and the level of measurements of the variables involved. Statistics of a single variable is always a descriptive statistics. If the data are numerical and normally distributed, we can use means and its standard deviation (standard error). If the distribution is not normal, we should use median (and relevant measures of dispersion). If the variable is categorical, we use proportion (percentage).
5. If we wish to study the association, we have basically two options: bivariable or multivariable analyses. When we are interested to study between just two variables, we choose the test based on level measurements, number of category (for categorical variable) and their distribution.
6. If we plan to study the relationship between three or more variables, we need suitable statistical tests such as linear regression, general linear model and logistic regression in SPSS. However, please take note that, just by running these tests does not mean that we are doing multivariate analysis because we can use them even for bivariable analyses. That is why we have simple linear regression or simple logistic regression. Simple denotes only one independent variable involved.
7. For any test chosen, it is important to take note the assumptions required.
8. Statistical tests are tools. Use them wisely and only choose the one that is relevant to achieve your objective.
9. One final note, always look beyond the numbers (given by the analysis). There many times clinical significance outweighs statistical significance.

Datasets

The following are list of datasets used in this book. Readers can download them from www.jamalrahman.net/book/dataset.

Data 1.1—Body weights
This set of data contains 100 random values of body weights in kg.

Data 2.1—High blood pressure
A study among 150 adults to measure the prevalence of high blood pressure and to describe any factors that may be associated with it. The variables include age (in years), gender, average income per month (RM), smoking status, body mass index (BMI) (kg/m2), fasting blood glucose (mmol/L) and fasting total cholesterol (mmol/L).

Data 2.2—Weight management programme
This data consist of 150 subjects whom blood pressure were tested before and after 6 months weight management programme. Their weight (in kg) and blood pressure status before and after the intervention were recorded.

Data 2.3—Waiting time
This is a study on waiting times (in minutes) among 80 patients who attended outpatient clinics divided into Medical and Surgical Units in three different settings (primary care, specialist and tertiary).

Data 2.4—Diabetic control and hypertension
A study on diabetic control (HbA1c in %) of 60 patients and its relationship with systolic blood pressure (SBP) (mmHg).

Data 2.5—Diabetic control and physical activity
A study to determine the relationship of physical activity measured in total weekly energy expenditure from leisure time physical activities for each individual in metabolic equivalents-hours (MET-Hr) for 58 diabetic patients. Diabetic control was measured using HbA1c (%). Confounders include age, sex and BMI (kg/m2).

J. Ab Rahman, *Brief Guidelines for Methods and Statistics in Medical Research*, SpringerBriefs in Statistics,
DOI 10.1007/978-981-287-925-7

Data 2.6—Factor affecting systolic blood pressure
A study to determine factors that affecting systolic blood pressure (SBP) among 75 adults. Factors being studied are age (in years), daily calories (0=Within recommended dietary allowance (RDA); 1=Above RDA) and physical activity level (0=Low, 1=Moderate and 2=High).

Data 2.7—Biomaterial versus autograft in fractured long bone
Bone lost during fracture is common. The gold standard to manage bone lost is using autologous bone graft harvested usually from iliac crest to fill in the gap. Recently, there are already many new biomaterials that can substitute or can be used in conjunction with patient's own bone graft. Some studies showed that the combination of biomaterial with platelet can increase efficacy. A trial was conducted among 80 patients who sustained fracture of long bones (humerus, tibia or femur) to compare the effectiveness of this biomaterial and biomaterial plus platelet versus autograft. The outcome measured was the total hospital cost ($) and the length of stay (days). Age of patients was recorded as a possible confounder apart from the site of fracture mentioned above.

Data 2.8—Blood sugar control
This is a study to measure the effect of low sugar diet in managing diabetic patients. All patients have comparable sex and age; received same medication and had their fasting blood sugar measured daily for 4 days.

Data 2.9—Obstructive sleep apnoea
A cross-sectional study was done in one primary school involving 109 students aged 7–12 years old. All students undergone polysomnography (sleep study) to detect the presence of obstructive sleep apnoea (OSA) coded 0=No, 1=Yes. Other variables include age (in years), gender (0=Female, 1=Male) and BMI status (categorised into 0=Normal, 1=Overweight and 2=Obese based on BMI for age).

References

Azmi Jr, M.Y., Junidah, R., Siti Mariam, A., Safiah, M.Y., Fatimah, S., Norimah, A.K., Poh, B.K., Kandiah, M., Zalilah, M.S., Wan Abdul Manan, W., Siti Haslinda, M.D., Tahir, A.: Body Mass Index (BMI) of adults: findings of the Malaysian Adult Nutrition Survey (MANS). Malays. J. Nutr. **15**(2), 97–119 (2009)

Department of Statistics Malaysia (2014) Concepts and definitions. http://www.statistics.gov.my/. Accessed 21 Jan 2014

Dupont, W.D., Plummer Jr, W.D.: Power and sample size calculations: a review and computer program. Control. Clin. Trials **11**(2), 116–128 (1990). doi:10.1016/0197-2456(90)90005-M

Fisher, R.A.: Statistical Methods for Research Workers. Cosmo Publications, New Delhi (1925)

Hill, A.B.: The environment and disease: association or causation? Proc. R. Soc. Med. **58**(5), 295–300 (1965)

Hill, A.B.: A Short Textbook of Medical Statistics. J. B. Lippincott Company, Philadelphia (1977)

Killip, S., Mahfoud, Z., Pearce, K.: What is an intracluster correlation coefficient? Crucial concepts for primary care researchers. Ann. Fam. Med. **2**(3), 204–208 (2004). doi:10.1370/afm.141

Kish, L.: Survey Sampling. Wiley, New York (1965)

Levine, T.R., Hullett, C.R.: Eta squared, partial eta squared, and misreporting of effect size in communication research. Hum. Commun. Res. **28**(4), 612–625 (2002). doi:10.1111/j.1468-2958.2002.tb00828.x

Olson, C.L.: Comparative robustness of six tests in multivariate analysis of variance. J. Am. Stat. Assoc. **69**(348), 894–908 (1974). doi:10.2307/2286159

Organization WH, Group ISoHW: 2003 World Health Organization (WHO)/International Society of Hypertension (ISH) statement on management of hypertension. J. Hypertens. **21**(11), 1983–1992 (2003)

Pierce, C.A.: Cautionary note on reporting eta-squared values from multifactor ANOVA designs. Educ. Psychol. Measur. **64**(6), 916–924 (2004). doi:10.1177/0013164404264848

VanVoorhis, C.R.W., Morgan, B.L.: Understanding power and rules of thumb for determining sample sizes. Tutorials Quant. Methods Psychol. **3**(2), 43–50 (2007)

J. Ab Rahman, *Brief Guidelines for Methods and Statistics in Medical Research*, SpringerBriefs in Statistics,
DOI 10.1007/978-981-287-925-7

Index

J. Ab Rahman, *Brief Guidelines for Methods and Statistics in Medical Research*, SpringerBriefs in Statistics,
DOI 10.1007/978-981-287-925-7

Printed in the United States
By Bookmasters

Printed in the United States
By Bookmasters